yoga
for a
new you

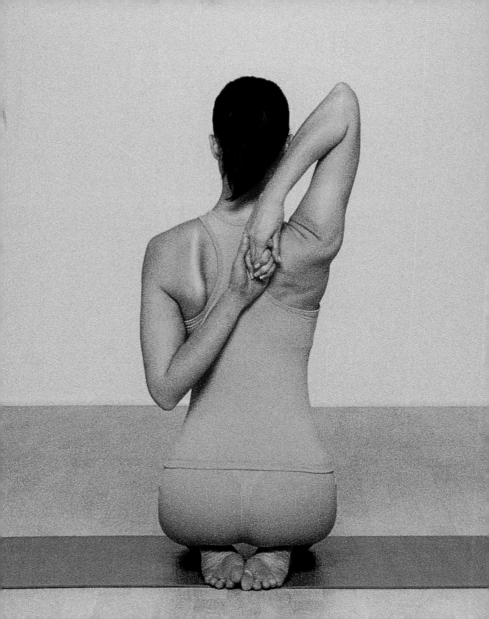

yoga
for a
new you

LONDON, NEW YORK, MUNICH,
MELBOURNE, AND DELHI

This revised edition
Project editor: Kathryn Meeker
Project designer: Charlotte Johnson
Managing editor: Penny Smith
Managing art editor: Marianne Markham
DTP designer: Sonia Charbonnier
Production editor: Siu Chan
Production controller: Seyhan Esen
Category publisher: Peggy Vance

Original editions
Series art editor: Anne-Marie Bulat
Series editor: Jane Laing
Series consultant: Peter Falloon-Goodhew
Managing editor: Gillian Roberts
Senior art editor: Karen Sawyer
Category publisher: Mary-Clare Jerram
Production controller: Joanna Bull
Photographer: Graham Atkins-Hughes (represented
by A & R Associates)

Material first published in the United States in Yoga For Living:
Feel Confident (2002), Yoga For Living: Boost Energy (2002),
Yoga For Living: Stay Young (2002), and Yoga for Living:
Relieve Stress (2002).

First American Edition, 2012
Published in the United States by
DK Publishing
375 Hudson Street
New York, New York 10014

12 13 14 15 10 9 8 7 6 5 4 3 2 1

001—183095—January/2012

Color reproduction by Media Development Printing Ltd.
Printed and bound in China by Hung Hing

Discover more at **www.dk.com**

contents

introduction

The holistic practices of yoga work on the physical, mental, emotional, and spiritual planes, enabling you to relieve stress, boost energy levels, feel more confident, and look and feel younger for longer.

The appeal of yoga is universal and timeless. Its combination of physical postures, breathing practices, relaxation, meditation, and lifestyle guidance is a tried-and-tested practical method of achieving all-around good health. Yoga does not seek to offer a quick fix, but provides a long-term program for living positively and mindfully.

For many people yoga becomes a life-long journey of self-discovery, bringing peace of mind and inner happiness. Unlike many forms of exercise, yoga is suitable for everyone. It is not competitive like most other aspects of life; you work with yourself as you are. Regular practice develops self-acceptance, which in turn leads to personal growth. Whatever your age or level of fitness, yoga is a safe form of exercise for everyone, provided you work within your limits.

About the book
Yoga for a New You consists of four sections: *Relaxed*, *Energetic*, *Young*, and *Confident*. Each section offers advice, techniques, postures, and programs that will guide you and help you achieve your goals.

Relaxed will show you ways to relieve stress and focus with quiet, easy-paced yoga techniques that decrease anxiety and help you respond effectively to the ups and downs of everyday life. Here yoga's holistic practices will allow you to reconnect with your real self and develop an inner calm and balance that enable you to manage stress effectively. By learning to observe the body objectively you can become truly aware of how you feel, and more able to understand what is happening in times of stress.

Energetic has practical yoga techniques and programs to harness mental and physical energy, boosting your stamina and enabling you to effectively manage your life and to live more positively. Sometimes energy becomes blocked, resulting in low levels of energy or an imbalance between physical, mental, and emotional energies. The central purpose of yoga is to enable us to experience the limitless life-energy that is the core of our being.

Young will help you tone, strengthen, and improve posture and mental agility with gentle techniques that promote a flexible mind and body. *Young* will help you to live more actively and mindfully, allowing you to retain your vitality and stay young at heart as you get older. Yoga can guide you to make changes that will help maintain a youthful outlook on life and give you peace of mind.

Confident explains how certain yoga postures can mobilize your core strength, and help you achieve mental clarity and face any situation with dignity and grace. It will help you to develop self-awareness on a physical, mental, and emotional level. Such awareness offers liberation from low self-esteem and a firm foundation on which to build self-confidence. Yoga promotes confidence and assuredness, allowing you to be comfortable and at ease with yourself. It gives unlimited access to the relaxed and respectful understanding that underpins self-confidence.

How yoga can help

Yoga for a New You will help you to develop a positive relationship with the world and with yourself, allowing life-energy to flow more freely through you. Through the practice of yoga you will learn how to slow down and get back in touch with the natural rhythms of your body, mind, and spirit. It will allow you to maintain a sensitive awareness of how things actually are, and what you really want out of life.

before
you start

Always try to practice yoga in the right spirit. Following the general guidance given here will help you practice with awareness and respect for your body's strengths and weaknesses.

Try to make a particular "time for me" every day to practice yoga. A few minutes every day is better than a whole hour once or twice a week.

Always practice on an empty stomach. Allow three hours to elapse after a large meal, two hours after a light meal, and one hour after a snack before starting your yoga practice. Wear comfortable clothes that do not restrict your movement or breathing. Practice on a mat or other nonslip surface, and make sure you have enough space around you to extend.

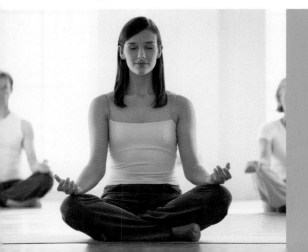

JOINING A CLASS

Practicing yoga regularly in a class with the expert guidance of an experienced yoga teacher can be invaluable when building self-confidence. Making such a commitment can help you develop your skills and abilities, and enhance the qualities of relaxation and ease. In addition, mutual respect between student and teacher promotes self-esteem.

Act "kindly" toward yourself as you practice. Looking after yourself is very important. Never push the body into discomfort or strain, as this is counterproductive. To begin with, you may feel some stiffness for a day or two, but it should soon pass.

Support from a teacher

When you are learning to manage stress, you will find it easier if you make a commitment to attend a regular suitable yoga class. You will need to check in your local area to find the right sort of class for you. Organizations that can help are listed on p.495. There are many different styles available. Some emphasize physical movement and postures; some are more meditative in type.

It is hard to overestimate the value of expert guidance from a qualified yoga teacher. You may want to take up the option of beginning with some individual classes with a qualified yoga therapist before you join a general class. If you want to begin to practice at home between classes, your teacher will be able to advise you what to do.

YOGA AND COMMON MEDICAL CONDITIONS

• If you have high blood pressure (HBP), a heart condition, glaucoma, or a detached retina, do not let your head stay below your heart.

• If you have HBP or a heart condition, hold strong standing and prone postures for a short time only. In addition, for HBP, keep your arms below your head.

• If you have low blood pressure (LBP), come up slowly from inverted poses.

• If you have a back problem or sciatica, avoid bending and twisting movements that provoke pain or other symptoms (for example, tingling or numbness in the leg). Keep your knees bent in forward bends.

• If you have a hernia, or have had recent abdominal surgery, do not put strong pressure on the abdomen.

• If you have arthritis, mobilize joints to their maximum pain-free range, but rest them if they are inflamed.

• If you have arthritis of the neck or other neck problems, do not tilt the head back in backbends and be cautious with sideways and twisting neck movements.

• During menstruation, energy levels may be lower than usual, and you may need to practice more gently. Avoid inversions and postures that put strong pressure on the pelvic area.

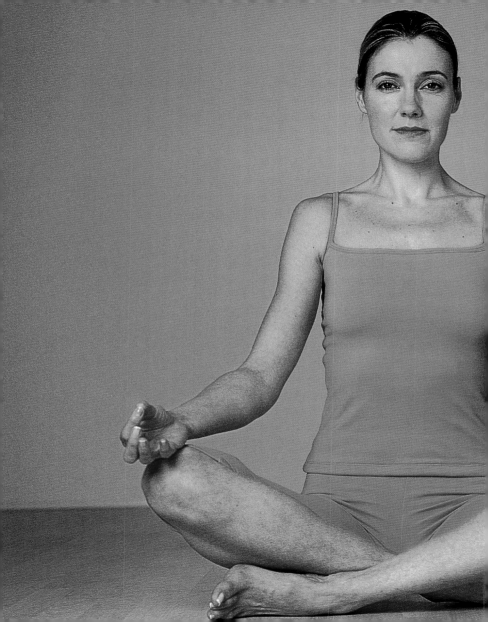

relaxed

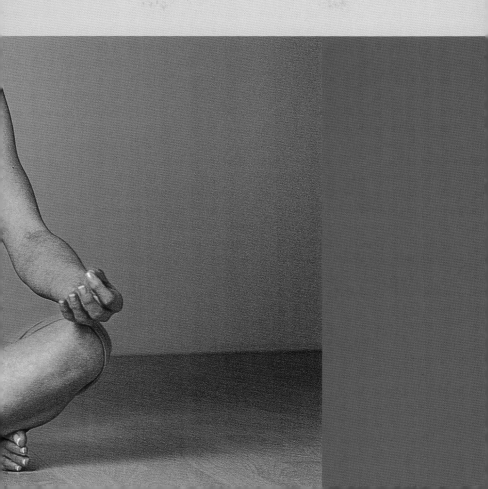

being
relaxed

The appeal of yoga is universal and timeless. Its holistic practices allow you to reconnect with your real self and develop an inner calm and balance that enable you to manage stress effectively.

Your body can tolerate enormous variation in living conditions, including extremes of temperature, humidity, and altitude. It is made up of millions of cells, organized into complex organs and systems, which cooperate with one another to provide a stable internal environment in which the cells can survive, whatever is going on in the outside world.

Throughout life, the body continually responds to events and activities as required. Whether you are asleep, exercising, or even standing on your head, the body will adjust your heart rate, blood pressure, and breathing to maintain this all-important internal stability.

Any factor that threatens to overwhelm or destabilize this balance is called a stressor, and the resulting effect on the body is known as stress. Stressors can affect the body in different ways. Physical stressors

HEALTH CONCERNS

If a health practitioner has advised you not to over-exert yourself physically, or if you have any other health concerns, seek advice from a qualified yoga therapist or teacher (see p.495) before using this book. Page 9 provides basic advice for some common medical conditions and, where appropriate, "Take Care" advice and "Alternatives" are given for individual practices. If you are pregnant, or have recently given birth, ask a suitably qualified yoga teacher which practices would be appropriate for you.

include extremes of climate and altitude, bodily injury, exercise, and lack of sleep. Psychological factors, such as fear, grief, and anxiety, also activate the stress response.

Positive stressors

Not all stressors are detrimental to the body. We need a certain amount of stimulation to stay healthy and active. Children who are deprived of play with others and who receive little or no cuddling often become adults with physical, behavioral, and psychological problems. Stressors provide stimulus, without which our minds and bodies would sink into inertia and depression.

The right amount of stress can actually enhance performance. Most public performers recognize the benefit of just enough "stage nerves," and sports people know the importance of the "adrenalin rush" in enabling them to compete to the best of their ability.

Enjoyable events and activities may also trigger stress responses. Research has shown that getting married or going on vacation can be almost as stressful as losing your job or moving home.

For optimum, all-around health you need to experience the right amount of the right types of stressors. In addition, you need to know how to cope with stressor overload or with exposure to unpleasant stressors.

Acute and chronic stress

Stress can be acute or chronic. Our bodies are designed to be able to deal with an acutely stressful situation by activating the "fright, fight, or flight" (FFF) reaction. FFF is a reflex multisystem response produced by the sympathetic part of the nervous system. It prepares the body for the possible need to either fight or run away from danger.

The rate and depth of breathing increases. The heart rate rises, while the heart pumps more strongly. Blood is quickly redirected to the brain and muscles, and away from areas such as the skin and digestive tract, where normal function can be safely suspended during the emergency. The pupils dilate to be able to see better, and the whole body is put on a state of alert by the outpouring of the hormone adrenalin from the adrenal glands into the circulation. Adrenalin production also affects the secretion of many other hormones, coordinating the multisystem effect.

When the acute situation is over, the FFF reaction dies away. The normal state of balance is restored quite quickly, and any sense of reaction or tiredness soon disappears.

Regular exposure to too many stressors produces a more chronic state of affairs, with the FFF reaction remaining partially and continuously activated. In this state, adrenalin levels in the blood are higher than normal, and the individual feels constantly on edge, gradually less and less able to cope, and more and more exhausted.

Negative stressors

Stressors can affect the body, the mind, and the spirit. The body is put under stress if you live in a harsh environment, with marked swings of temperature and humidity, or at high altitude. Fortunately, most of us do not have this problem.

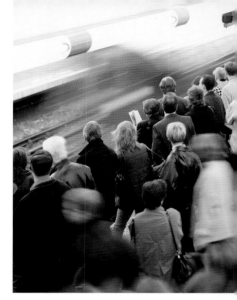

Facing the rush-hour crush morning and evening every weekday can increase your physical stress levels considerably.

Many of us do regularly experience less extreme physical stressors, such as exposure to city air pollution and environmental toxins. Uncomfortable working conditions, such as poorly designed seating or working night shifts, also affect significant numbers of people, as does crowded and unreliable public transportation.

Mental stresses are more common than physical ones. Today's high-tech communication systems have contributed to the development of a faster pace of life than humankind has experienced in its entire history. Leisure time – "time for me" – can be almost impossible to find, and when a break does present itself, you may find that you have become unable to switch off and relax.

The experience of chronic stress can lead over time to a sense of dis-spiritedness. It is easy nowadays to feel that you are on a treadmill, with no respite from the daily grind.

Being in such a situation can lead to psychological illnesses, such as anxiety and depression. The effect of high levels of stress hormones, such as adrenalin and cortisol, disrupts normal physiological functions, leaving the body vulnerable to a host of physical ailments. High blood pressure, infections, allergies, skin rashes, and digestive problems are only some of the conditions made worse by chronic overstress.

Factors affecting stress levels

Modern lifestyles certainly contribute to the buildup of chronic stress. Most people work, either as employees or in self-employment. Many employees

SIGNS OF OVERSTRESS

Chronic overstress produces numerous physical, mental, and emotional signs.

• Muscle tension in the neck and shoulders causes pain and stiffness.

• Muscle tension in the scalp and jaw results in headaches and face pain. Migraines are common, as are episodes of teeth grinding at night, nail biting, fidgeting, and foot tapping.

• The heart beats faster, the breathing becomes shallow, and you sweat.

• Digestive problems produce heartburn, irritable bowel syndrome (IBS), and bowel disturbances.

• You feel driven and under constant pressure. You suffer tiredness, anxiety, depression, continual worrying, and an overactive mind that is never still.

• Attacks of insomnia add an overlying element of physical tiredness, while the inability to switch off upsets sleep patterns even more.

• Panic attacks may occur, stimulating the release of even more adrenaline. The appetite can become disturbed, and increased alcohol intake can lead to alcohol dependence.

• Smoking, which many use in an attempt to de-stress, only makes matters worse by saturating the body with toxins and damaging the lungs and blood vessels.

are subject to regular performance scrutiny, with deadlines and sales targets to achieve. Salaries may contain a bonus element that can be acquired only through extra working hours. For those in management, added responsibilities increase the pressure.

Many people, especially women, are "multitasking," juggling careers with home and family responsibilities in addition to work commitments. This can require an almost super-human ability to plan, prioritize, and carry out numerous tasks, usually several at once. No wonder many women feel that during the years spent raising their families they are always tired, and always cross!

Lifestyle events can produce unbearable stressors. Events such as bereavement, divorce, moving home, having a baby, and changing jobs each result in considerable stress. If more than one of these significant events occurs within a short period, you may well become overstressed.

Many of us lead sedentary lives. Sometimes this is by choice, but often it is because we just cannot find the time to exercise. The body is designed to be used: without regular exercise it becomes stiff and weak.

Equally, too much exercise can be as stressful as too little. Exercise addiction, in which the body is pushed to its limits too often, has become some people's way of coping with stress. This may be connected with the desire to look like a celebrity role model, but it reveals a deep inner dissatisfaction. Unfortunately, the overall effect is to increase stress levels, not reduce them.

You can unwittingly increase your stress level by adopting poor standing and sitting postures. Sitting for long periods at work or in the car does not help; nor does standing and walking, carrying shopping bags, school bags, or toddlers, especially all at once. Such physical stressors can cause pain and tension in the neck, shoulders, and lower back.

Your mental or emotional state can affect your stress levels markedly. When faced with forthcoming examinations or an interview, you can put so much pressure on yourself to do well that you overstress yourself.

Medical conditions, especially those causing pain or chronic discomfort, increase stress levels in the sufferer. Arthritis, ME, fibromyalgia, irritable bowel syndrome, and similar conditions can make the everyday tasks of life more difficult to perform, adding to the pressure.

Modern global communications mean that most people become aware of natural and man-made disasters almost as soon as they happen, even when they are thousands of miles away. Graphic images and heart-rending interviews act as marked stressors, especially when you feel powerless to do anything.

Restoring the balance

When you are being bombarded by numerous stressors, you must review your lifestyle and determine to change it where necessary. However, before you can change the way you live, you must become aware of how you actually feel. Stress can mask the information being sent to the brain

by the thousands of sensory nerve endings situated all over the body. In this way, you progressively lose touch with yourself. Consequently, you do not notice tiredness until it becomes exhaustion, or muscle tension until it becomes unbearable.

When you reach this point, it is imperative that you learn how to slow down, to get back in touch with the natural rhythms of the body,

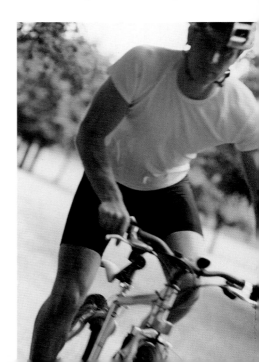

Incorporating regular exercise, such as bicycling, into your routine helps keep you fit and more able to deal with stress.

mind, and spirit. By learning to observe the body objectively, you can become truly aware of how you feel, and more able to understand what is happening at times because of stress.

When you are able to really get in touch with yourself, the symptoms of stress begin to reduce. Panic attacks, and other manifestations of stress, subside, and you feel they are no longer controlling you.

How can yoga help?

Yoga is the age-old lifestyle system that reconnects you with your real self. It then maintains that sensitive awareness of how things actually are, and what you really want out of life. Yoga works at all levels of the individual – through the body, mind, and spirit simultaneously.

Gentle, enjoyable stretches and asanas (traditional yoga postures) ease out muscle tensions and limber the joints, while at the same time maintaining the general health of

the body. Relaxation techniques further help the body let go of tension and become re-energized.

In yoga, working with the breath is an integral part of the practice – the breath acts as a link between the body and mind. Simple breathing practices encourage quietness of mind and teach the "thinking" parts of the mind to relax and rest. These

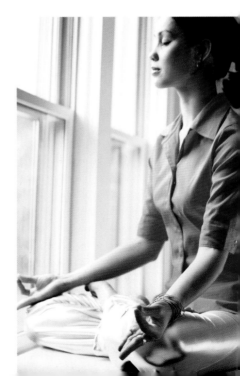

Simple breathing practices, using a mudra (symbolic hand gesture), can help you to centre yourself, restoring peace of mind and inner calm during stressful situations.

practices lead to the development of simple meditation, which deepens the experience of inner calm. This sense of tranquility and balance is then carried into everyday life to enable you to manage and do well in the most stressful situations.

Unlike most other aspects of life, yoga is noncompetitive; you work with yourself as you are. Regular practice develops self-acceptance, which in turn leads to personal growth. Many other stress-relieving practices, such as reflexology and massage, although valuable, require someone else to provide the service; with yoga, you take responsibility for yourself and your practice.

As you become accustomed to regular yoga practice, you will find you begin to live yoga on a daily basis. Your whole attitude to life changes; you no longer find yourself exasperated by the habits or actions of colleagues or family members. You are able to stay calm when events do not work out as you hoped, and you are much more able to cope with day-to-day problems and find satisfactory solutions.

HOW TO USE THIS SECTION

Relaxed is divided into three sub-sections. **Foundations** provides guidance on practicing yoga and some basic breathing and preliminary stretches. Familiarize yourself with these first before moving on to **Building Blocks**. This contains a selection of postures and breathing practices, as well as a simple meditation and relaxation technique. Work through these postures gradually, selecting one or two to work on at a time, rather than trying to do them all in one session. Look at the photographs first to get a feel for the shape of the posture. Then follow the accompanying step-by-step instructions. If you find a posture difficult, work on the preliminary steps first or try the alternative, if one is given.

Programs combines selected postures and other practices in a series of short yoga programs designed for particular situations and needs. Make sure you understand how to do the postures first before trying these programs.

Yoga is traditionally learned from a teacher, and you will benefit from going to a class, if you are not already doing so. Organizations that can help you find a qualified teacher are listed on page 495.

the basics

In yoga, basic standing, sitting, and lying-down positions are important in their own right, helping you develop stability and awareness of the benefits of alignment for your posture and breathing, and for the free flow of energy. They also provide the foundations on which other postures are developed.

In addition, being able to sit comfortably and steadily is important for breathing practices and also for meditation, helping you remain focused without distractions from physical tensions. Lying down is often used to develop body and breath awareness, and to relax and allow

your body to absorb the beneficial effects of other yoga practices.

If you find it impossible to achieve the full posture, it can be very helpful to use a prop, such as a block or cushion, to make sure you do not strain your body.

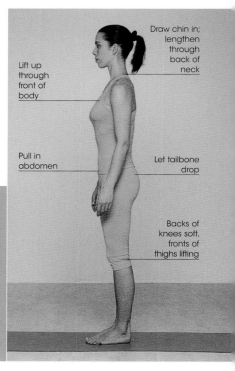

Lift up through front of body

Draw chin in; lengthen through back of neck

Pull in abdomen

Let tailbone drop

Backs of knees soft, fronts of thighs lifting

STANDING

Stand up straight with your feet parallel, hip-width apart, and your ears, tops of shoulders, hips, and ankles in line. Press your feet into the ground and lift up through your body. Broaden across the top of the chest. Feel balanced in every direction, as if your head is suspended by a thread from the ceiling. Look straight ahead, relax, and breathe easily.

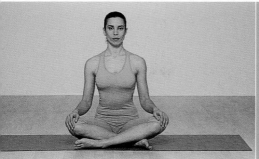

SITTING CROSS-LEGGED

This posture is good for breathing practices. Cross your shins with the feet under the opposite knee. Position yourself on the front edge of your sitting bones, with the spine long and the head erect. Relax the shoulders. If your knees are higher than your hips, sit on a block.

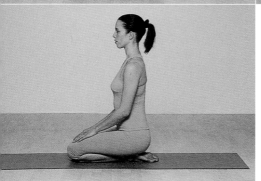

KNEELING

If you find sitting cross-legged uncomfortable, try kneeling. Sit on your heels with the tops of your thighs facing the ceiling. Or position your knees and feet hip-width apart and sit on blocks, a folded blanket, or a bolster. Keep your spine long and your head erect, the shoulders and neck relaxed.

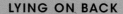

LYING ON BACK

Lie with your legs stretched out, hip-width apart. Relax the legs, and allow the feet and legs to roll out. Place your arms away from the body, the backs of the hands on the floor. Relax the neck and rest the center of the back of the head on the floor.

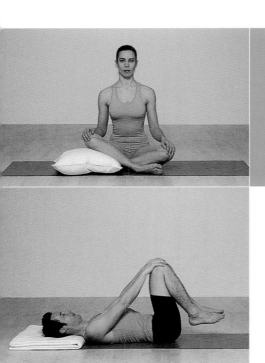

USING A PILLOW

Pillows can be used to support different parts of the body. Here one is shown supporting the thigh while sitting cross-legged. This allows the inner and the outer thigh muscles to relax and the hips to open farther, helping the student to stay in the posture longer without being distracted by discomfort.

USING A BLANKET

When lying supine, the back of the neck should be long, with the chin a little down toward the chest, and not pointing up to the ceiling. If you find it difficult to keep the neck long, place a folded blanket under the head and neck for additional support.

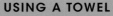

USING A TOWEL

Kneeling positions can put strain on stiff ankles. To relieve this, roll up a towel firmly and place it between the ankles and the floor. A folded towel can also be used under bony parts of the feet or ankles, especially if you are working on a hard floor.

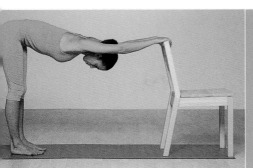

USING A CHAIR

Chairs can be used to modify postures. Shown here is a version of the Forward Bend. You can also use a chair for breathing or meditation practices if sitting or kneeling on the floor is uncomfortable. Sit toward the front of the chair, with the soles of the feet flat on the floor, hands on thighs.

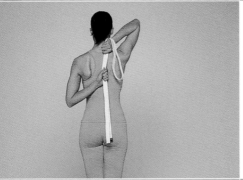

USING A BELT

A nonstretchy webbing belt or luggage strap can help you to release a stiff neck or tight shoulders. Looping a belt around the feet in some sitting postures, such as forward bends, can also help you lift the breastbone and lengthen the spine while keeping the shoulders relaxed.

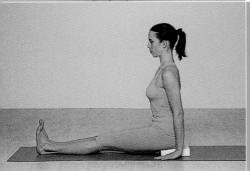

USING A FOAM BLOCK

A firm foam block will help if you find it difficult to lengthen the spine in sitting postures, as it optimizes the tilt of the pelvis. Sit toward the front of the block, not in the middle of it. If you do not have a block, use a telephone directory or small, firm cushion.

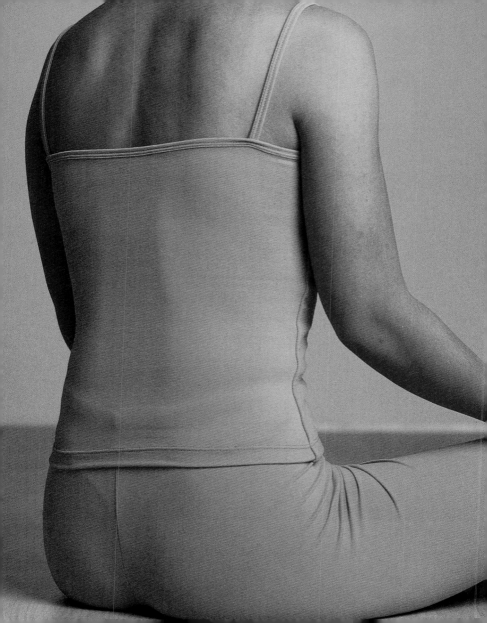

foundations

This section shows you some basic standing, sitting, and lying postures. It provides breath-with-movement exercises to loosen your body and help you deepen the connection with the breath. Breathing and centering techniques are given to bring awareness to your practice.

centering

Learning how to be centered is a fundamental aspect of yoga practice. It enables you to connect with your breath, becoming refreshed and re-energized from the quietness that lies within you.

In everyday life your attention is turned outward as you relate to the people and events around you. This can result in your energy being sapped, leaving you feeling tired and tense. The practice of centering enables you to balance your daily life with periods of quiet. You can practice centering lying on your back, sitting, or standing. Find somewhere quiet where you will not be disturbed, and make yourself comfortable.

becoming centered

1 If you choose to lie down, lie on your back, let your legs and feet roll out, and position your arms slightly away from your body. Keep the back of the neck long, drawing the chin gently down toward the chest. If you prefer to sit cross-legged or to stand, lift the breastbone a little and relax the shoulders.

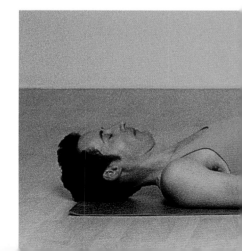

2 Close the eyes gently. Relax the scalp. Relax the face and release any tension in the jaw. Turn your attention inward, and get in touch with your body and how it feels. Begin to notice the gentle movement of the body with the breath. Feel the sensations within your body that result from these movements.

3 Be aware that you are not making the breath happen; neither are you controlling it in any way. Rather, you are trusting the body to breathe just as you do while you are asleep. Let your breath settle into a slow, deep, natural rhythm. Observe it flowing in and out of your body.

4 Let your attention be with your breath and the sensations in the body for a little while. You will find even a few breaths like this helpful, or you can practice for several minutes.

5 When you notice that your attention has wandered and you are thinking of something else, gently draw your awareness back to your breath, without analysis or judgment. It does not matter if your thoughts stray often at first. All you have to do is keep bringing your attention back to the breath each time it happens. The mind soon gets used to focusing lightly on the breath without strain. All it takes is a little practice.

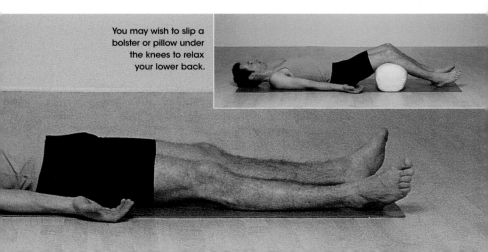

You may wish to slip a bolster or pillow under the knees to relax your lower back.

basic
breathing

There is a fundamental connection between the breath and your physical, mental, and emotional states. By working with the breath, you will be able to let go of stress in any situation.

Breathing provides oxygen for the metabolic processes from which we derive the energy to move, think, and feel, and carries away carbon dioxide, the main waste product of our metabolism. Physical tension in the respiratory muscles between and within the ribs can cause tightness in the chest, and even chest pain. Relaxed breathing techniques will release tension from the whole of the upper body, including the neck and shoulders. This will improve your ability to adjust your breathing to meet changing requirements.

The breath also provides a powerful link between mind and body. By controlling your breathing patterns – for example, the rhythm and depth of breathing, the length of the out-breath, and the balance between right and left nostrils – you can influence your physical, mental, and emotional states.

Good breathing habits

Yoga encourages breathing through the nose, full use of the diaphragm, a slow, smooth breathing pattern, and coordination of movement and breath. Opening movements, such as back bends, are practiced on an in-breath, and closing movements, such as forward bends, on the out-breath.

The breathing practice opposite will help develop awareness of the action of respiratory muscles and encourage good breathing habits. It can be done standing, lying down, or sitting as well as kneeling.

sitting sectional breathing

Sectional breathing helps release muscle tension associated with poor breathing habits. After completing

Step 3, combine all three steps to produce full, continuous in-breaths and out-breaths.

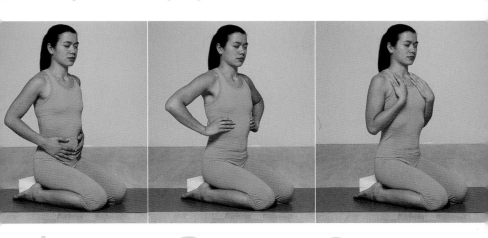

1 Kneel comfortably with your palms resting on your abdomen, the middle fingers just touching. Breathe into your hands, feeling the abdomen swell out and the fingers move apart as you breathe in. Then feel the abdomen sink back as you exhale. Take six even breaths.

2 Bring your hands to your ribcage, with your fingers to the front and thumbs on the back ribs. Feel the ribs expand into the hands on the in-breath and relax back inward as you exhale. Take six breaths, breathing into the sides of the chest.

3 Place your fingers on your collarbones, in front of your shoulders. Breathe in, feeling the fingers and shoulders rise up toward the head, and the top of the chest expand. As you breathe out, feel the fingers sink back down with the chest. Take six breaths.

breath with
movement

These simple postures are designed to deepen your connection with your breath as well as gently move your joints. Each movement is timed to match the length of the breath.

supine arms over head

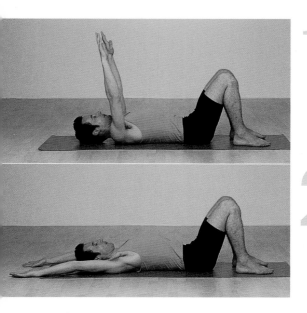

1 Lie with your knees bent and your feet on the floor. Place the feet and knees hip-width apart, arms alongside the body with the palms down. Connect with your breath. As you breathe in, bring the arms slowly and smoothly up and back behind the head.

2 Soften the elbows and relax the shoulders, so that the arms are on the floor behind your head by the time you have completed the in-breath. As you breathe out, slowly return the arms to the starting position alongside the body. Repeat for six to eight breaths.

supine nurturing

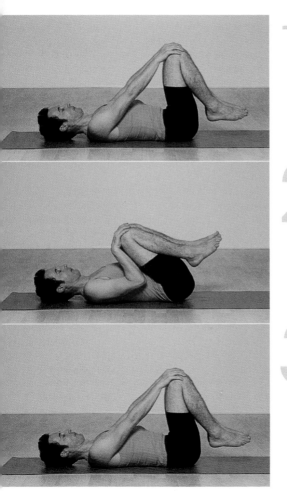

1 Lie on your back. Draw the knees up and place one hand on each kneecap, with the fingers pointing toward the feet, the knees together. Relax your shoulders. As you breathe in, send the knees away from you.

2 As you breathe out, draw the knees in toward the chest, bending your arms. Keep the shoulders relaxed and the neck long throughout.

3 As you breathe in, straighten your arms enough to send the knees away from you. Continue these movements, coordinated with the breath, for 10 to 12 breaths. This simple moving posture is one of the best for relieving stress. It also eases the back and hips when you have been sitting for long periods.

supine legs up arms out

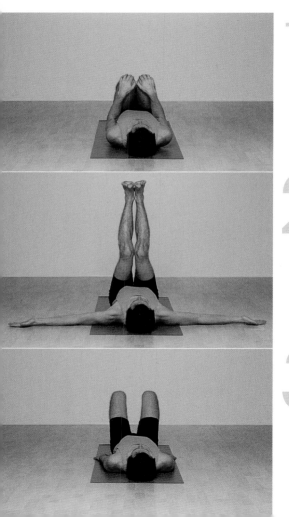

1 Lie on your back with the knees bent. Draw up the knees and place one hand over each kneecap, the fingers pointing toward the feet. Relax the shoulders and draw the chin a little down toward the chest, so that the back of the neck is long.

2 As you breathe in, take the arms out to the floor at shoulder height. At the same time, take the feet up toward the ceiling. Keep the feet together and the knees slightly bent.

3 As you breathe out, bring your legs back down slowly and place your hands on your kneecaps again. Repeat for six to eight breaths. Find a comfortable breathing rate and let your movements be governed by the breath. Then bring the feet to the floor, arms each side of the body.

supine twist

1 Lie with the knees bent, the feet together on the floor close to the hips. Position the arms away from the body at an angle of about 45 degrees. Relax the shoulders.

2 As you breathe out, slowly let the knees sink over to the left. Your hips will roll so you are now lying more on the left hip. Turn the head to the right. Relax the feet. As you breathe in, slowly return to the starting position.

3 As you breathe out, slowly let the knees sink over to the right, turning the head to the left. Keep the shoulders and feet relaxed. As you breathe in, slowly return to the starting position. Repeat the sequence for six to eight breaths. Feel the quietening effects as you work with the breath.

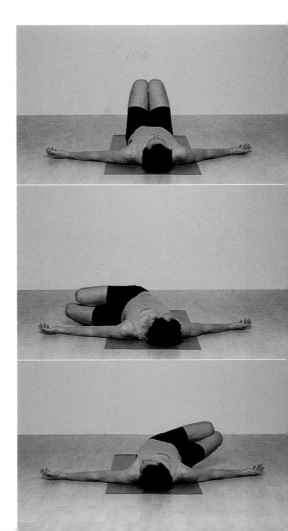

standing arm stretches

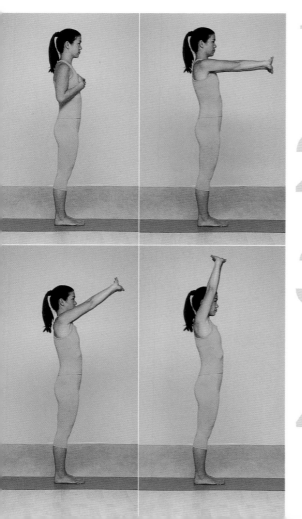

1 Stand, feet together. Become aware of the flow of the breath. Clasp your hands and place them over the breast bone. Keep the elbows and shoulders relaxed.

2 As you breathe in, turn the palms out and stretch them away from you, straightening the elbows. As you breathe out, return to the starting position. Repeat twice.

3 As you breathe in, turn the palms out and stretch them up away from you at an angle of 45 degrees, keeping the shoulders relaxed. As you breathe out, return to the starting position. Repeat twice.

4 As you breathe in, turn the palms away and stretch them right up vertically, keeping the shoulders relaxed. As you breathe out, return to the starting position. Repeat twice more, then unclasp the hands.

french press stretch

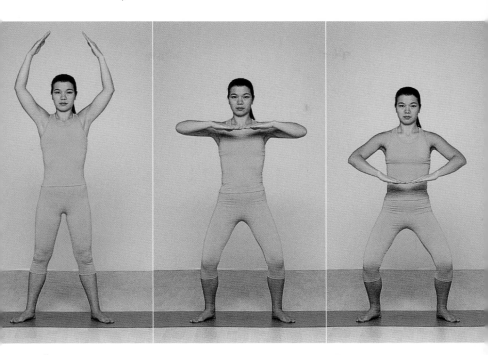

1 Stand with the feet more than hip-width apart and the toes turned out. As you breathe in, stretch the arms out to the sides, palms up, and circle them up to almost meet above your head.

2 Imagine you have in front of you a huge French press plunger. As you breathe out, bring your arms in front of your chest until your fingers touch. Bend slightly at the knees and begin to push down with your hands.

3 Continue to push down the imaginary plunger until your hands are level with your waist. Then repeat four to six times, coordinating the actions with the breathing.

neck stretches

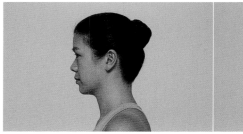

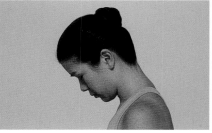

1 These gentle movements ease out muscle tension in the neck and shoulders. Sit cross-legged on the floor or on an upright chair. Lift the breastbone and relax the shoulders.

2 Allow the head to come forward slowly under its own weight, bringing the chin down toward the chest. Keep the breastbone up. Stay in this position for several breaths.

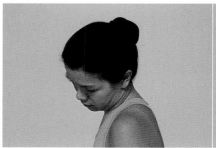

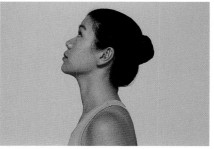

3 Allow the head to roll slowly to the left until the ear is over the shoulder. Stay for several breaths, then return to the midline position and repeat on the right. Return to the starting position.

4 Lift the chin slowly toward the ceiling, keeping the back of the neck long. Feel the stretch in all parts of the neck, hold for a few breaths, and return to the starting position.

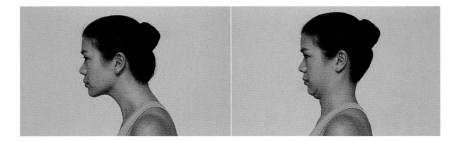

Looking straight ahead, slowly send the chin forward, keeping it parallel to the floor. Hold for a few breaths. Keep the shoulders relaxed throughout.

Slowly draw the chin back as far as you comfortably can, keeping it parallel to the floor. Hold for a few breaths, and then return to the starting position.

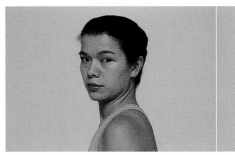

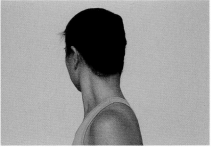

Keeping the shoulders relaxed, slowly turn the head to look over the left shoulder as far as you comfortably can. Hold for several breaths.

Return to the starting position, then turn the head to look over the right shoulder as far as you comfortably can. Hold for several breaths.

standing upward stretch

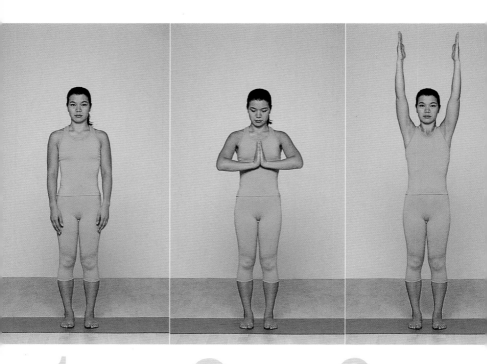

1 Stand with the feet parallel and a little apart. Rock a bit on your feet to balance your body weight evenly. Feel balanced and grounded, letting your weight pass into the floor.

2 Gently lift the kneecaps up a little, relax the shoulders, and lift up the breastbone. Bring the palms together in front of the heart. Look down at the floor past your hands.

3 Slowly stretch the arms up above your head, the palms facing one another. On an in-breath, lift up the chest and stretch. On the out-breath, bring the arms down and let them relax.

half forward bend

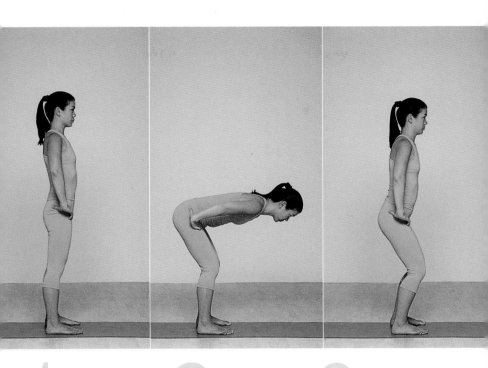

1 Stand with the feet hip-width apart, the inside edges of the feet parallel. Take your hands to the crease at the top of the leg, where the leg joins the body. Your hip joints lie behind your hands.

2 Lift the breastbone up away from the floor, to lengthen the front of the body. On an out-breath, stretch forward with a straight back until your upper body is parallel to the floor. Look down.

3 Bend the knees when you feel the stretch in the backs of the legs. Connect with your breath for several breaths. On an in-breath, come up slowly with knees bent, and return to Step 1.

standing back arch

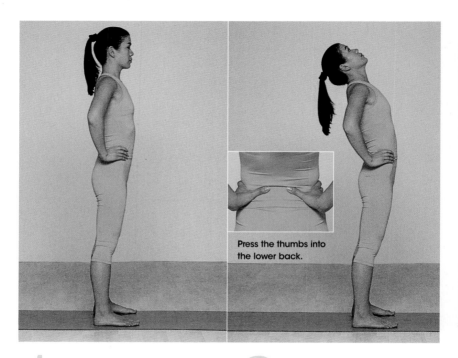

Press the thumbs into the lower back.

1 Stand with the feet hip-width apart and the inside edges of the feet parallel, the hands on the hips. Take the hands back a little, so the thumbs rest against the lower back, a few inches apart. Now roll the shoulders back to open up the chest. Tuck the chin in.

2 Begin to lift the breastbone up away from the floor. As you lift, feel the upper body arching back. Now lift the chin to look toward the ceiling and breathe for several breaths. Keep lifting the breastbone. Slowly release the pose by lifting the breastbone as you return to an upright position.

standing side stretch

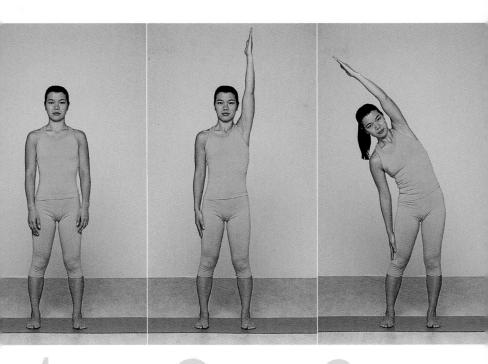

1. Stand with your feet parallel and hip-width apart, your arms down by your sides. If you have back problems, place your right hand on your hip.

2. As you breathe in, raise the left arm up beside your head, fingers reaching up to the ceiling, shoulders relaxed down away from the ears. Try to bring the raised arm to touch the left ear.

3. Reach up and out to the right on an out-breath. Hold, then return to an upright position on an in-breath. Circle the arm back down on the out-breath. Repeat on the other side.

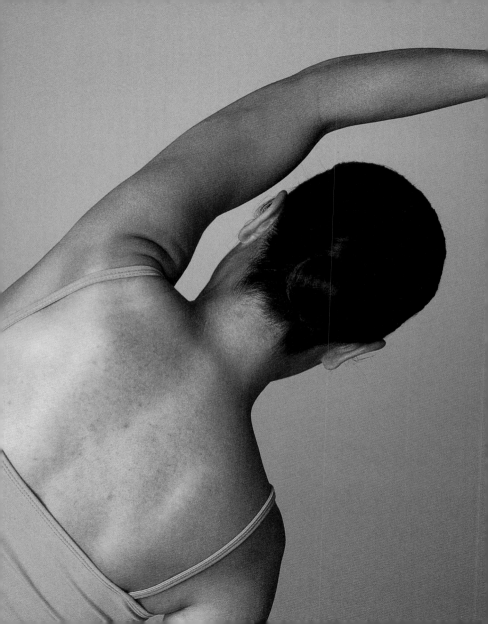

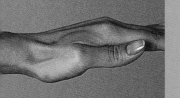

building blocks

This section presents a variety of postures and other yoga practices to calm body, mind, and spirit. Stay in the postures only for as long as you are able to hold them steadily and comfortably, breathing evenly. Listen to your body as you practice, and you will make steady progress.

eagle

This posture opens and stretches across the upper back, neck, and shoulders, releasing tension in these areas. The arms represent the eagle's folded wings and the fingers represent the feathers.

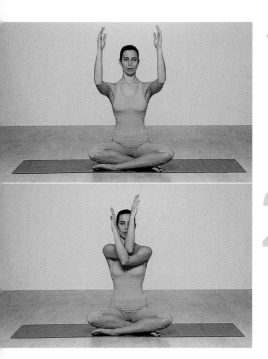

1 Sit cross-legged on the floor (use a foam block or small pillow, if necessary), hands on knees. Lift the breastbone and relax the shoulders. Bring both arms up in front of you, palms facing each other. Bend the elbows and hold them at shoulder height and shoulder-width apart, so each arm forms a right angle.

2 Lower the left elbow a little and send the left hand away from you slightly. As you breathe in, bring the arms toward and past each other, hooking the left elbow under the right one.

TAKE CARE
• If you have neck problems, tilt the head a little forward.
• If you have stiff shoulders, do not strain to achieve the final position.

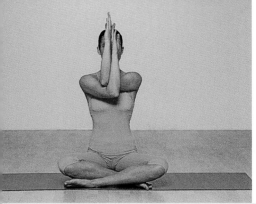

Breathing out, bring the backs of the forearms and the backs of the hands toward each other directly in front of your face. Bring them as close together as you can without straining your shoulders. Now let the breath flow in and out naturally.

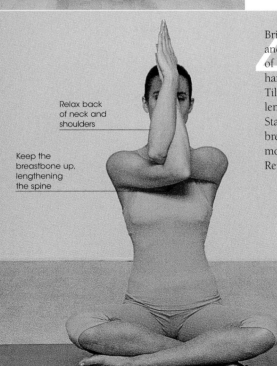

Relax back of neck and shoulders

Keep the breastbone up, lengthening the spine

Bring the left hand toward you and then slip it into the palm of the right, stretching the right-hand fingers toward the ceiling. Tilt the head a little forward to lengthen the back of the neck. Stay in the posture for several breaths, feeling the breath moving the back of the ribcage. Repeat on the other side.

COW

This posture stretches across the front of the body, opening the armpits and releasing tension in the neck and shoulders. As the breath is in the ribcage, the posture has an overall energizing effect.

1 Assume the basic kneeling position. Lift the breastbone and relax the shoulders. Take the left arm up the back, positioning the back of the hand between the shoulder blades, or as high as it will comfortably reach. To help position the left hand, reach behind you with the right hand and, holding onto the left elbow, draw it toward the trunk.

2 Breathing in, raise the right arm vertically. Lift the ribs on the right side of the chest, open the armpit, and stretch the hand to the ceiling.

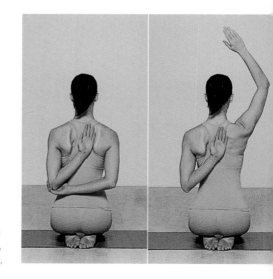

TAKE CARE
If you find one side easier than the other, practice the stiffer side before the "good" side, then repeat on the stiffer side again.

3 Bend the elbow of the right arm and lower the right hand down your back. Breathing out, hook the two hands together, then relax the neck. Hold the pose for several breaths, feeling the front of the ribcage moving with the breath. Release your hands and repeat with the left arm in the raised position.

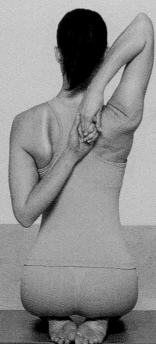

Front view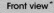

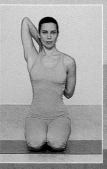

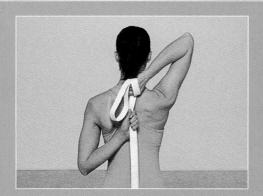

ALTERNATIVE

If the hands do not make contact, use a belt. Hold it in the right hand and lower it down behind you, reaching up for it with the left hand. When both hands are holding the belt, gather it in until the hands are comfortably close, and relax the neck.

forward
bend

Forward-stretching postures have a quietening effect on the mind. In the Forward Bend, you bend at the hips, keeping the back straight and the sitting bones lifting up to help release tight hamstrings.

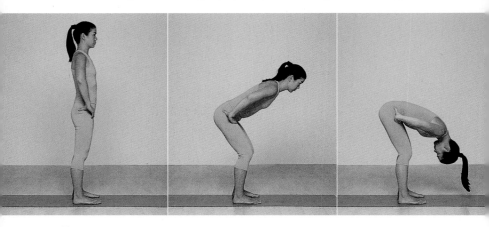

1 Stand with the feet hip-width apart and parallel. Take your hands to the crease at the tops of the legs at the point where they join the torso.

2 Lift the breastbone up away from the floor to lengthen the front of the body. As you breathe out, fold forward from the hips, bending slightly at the knees.

3 With your knees still bent, let the spine relax and lengthen as gravity pulls the head and upper body down toward the floor. Breathe easily.

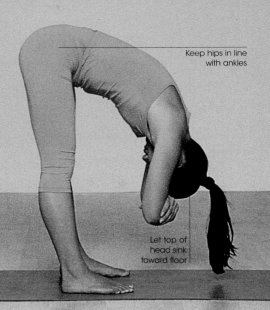

4 Letting the upper body hang from the hips, press the feet into the floor and lift your sitting bones up to lengthen through the backs of the legs. Bring your arms above your head, and hold onto your elbows. Stay in the position for several breaths, keeping the stretch through the backs of the legs.

Keep hips in line with ankles

Let top of head sink toward floor

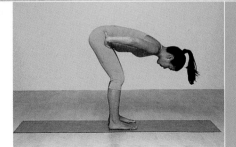

5 Bend your knees. Put your hands on your hips and come up halfway, lengthening through the upper spine. On an in-breath, come up to the basic standing position, hinging from the hips and keeping your back straight.

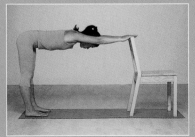

ALTERNATIVE

If you have HBP, glaucoma, or a detached retina, do a Half Forward Bend, resting your hands on the back of a chair. Keep the abdomen pulled back toward the spine and the chest lifted.

tree

In Tree, not only is the body balanced, but the mind becomes quiet and relaxed, too. This posture strengthens the leg muscles and promotes good alignment of the spine.

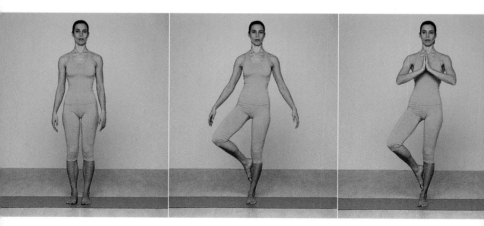

1 Stand up straight with your feet a little apart, your weight evenly distributed over both feet, and your arms by your sides.

2 Inhaling, bring the sole of the right foot against the inside of the standing leg just below the knee. Take the knee out to the side, to open the hip joint on that side.

3 As you breathe out, lift the breastbone up and relax the shoulders. Bring the palms together in front of your chest. Stop here if you have arthritis in the knees.

If you feel balanced, lift the foot and place the sole against the top of the inside of the standing leg. Breathing in, stretch your arms up above the head, keeping the palms together. Relax the shoulders and the face. To stay balanced, fix your gaze on a vertical line, such as the edge of a door. Breathe easily for several breaths, then release the pose. Pause and repeat on the other side.

TAKE CARE

If bringing the palms together creates tension in the neck or shoulders, keep the hands shoulder-width apart above the head.

Make sure fronts of both hips face directly forward

Take knee back without twisting hips

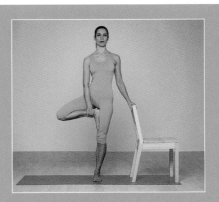

ALTERNATIVE

If your balance is poor, stand against a wall for support or hold onto the back of a chair, as shown. Holding the ankle of the raised leg may also be helpful.

side
warrior

This standing posture not only strengthens the body, but also enables you to become aware of the boundless reserves of inner strength that lie within you. Stay balanced and focused throughout.

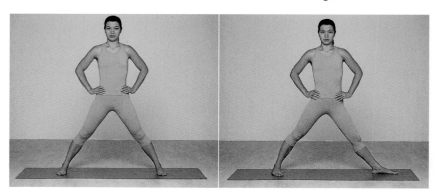

1 Stand with your feet about 3 ft (1 m) apart, the inside edges of the feet parallel, your hands on your waist, and your shoulders relaxed. Look straight ahead.

2 As you breathe in, turn the toes of the right foot in a little and turn all of the left leg out from the hip 90 degrees. Keep your upper body facing front.

TAKE CARE

- If you have HBP or a heart condition, hold for a short time only.
- Proceed cautiously if you have back problems.

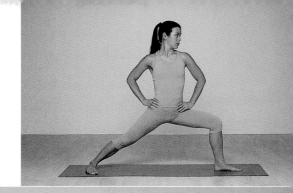

Breathing out, bend the left knee and let your hips sink toward the floor. Align the knee with the ankle to make a right angle with the leg. Turn your head to the left, but keep the shoulders facing the front.

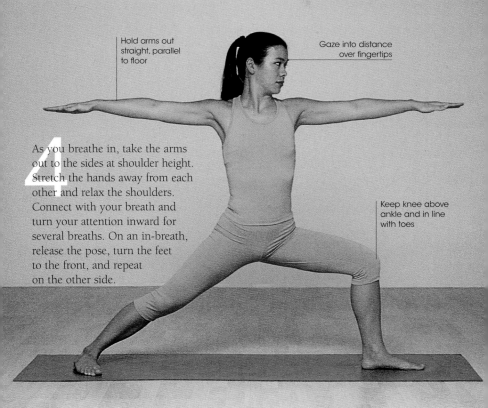

Hold arms out straight, parallel to floor

Gaze into distance over fingertips

As you breathe in, take the arms out to the sides at shoulder height. Stretch the hands away from each other and relax the shoulders. Connect with your breath and turn your attention inward for several breaths. On an in-breath, release the pose, turn the feet to the front, and repeat on the other side.

Keep knee above ankle and in line with toes

lunge
warrior

Lunge Warrior provides a powerful stretch through the back of the leg, thigh, and hip, extends the spine, and opens the chest. Feel the energy building as you breathe deeply into the ribcage.

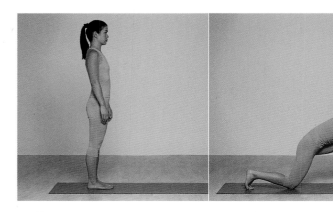

1 Stand up straight, feet hip-width apart, arms by your sides. Move onto all fours, keeping your toes curled under. Place your hands beneath the shoulders and knees beneath the hips.

2 As you exhale, take your left leg forward between your hands, so that your knee is directly above the heel of your left foot. Rest your upper body on the left thigh. Press your fingertips into the floor.

TAKE CARE
If you have back problems, do not go beyond Step 2 to begin with.

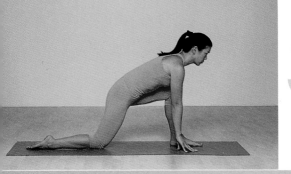

Keeping your fingers steepled, raise your head a little to look slightly farther ahead. Untuck the toes of your right foot, so that the top of the foot is resting on the floor.

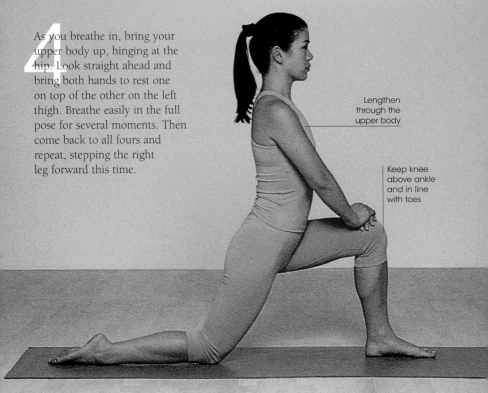

As you breathe in, bring your upper body up, hinging at the hip. Look straight ahead and bring both hands to rest one on top of the other on the left thigh. Breathe easily in the full pose for several moments. Then come back to all fours and repeat, stepping the right leg forward this time.

Lengthen through the upper body

Keep knee above ankle and in line with toes

downward dog

One of the great classical yoga postures, Downward Dog works and stretches the whole body, releasing tension and quietening the mind as it balances the upper and lower body.

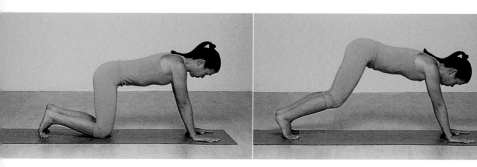

1 Begin on all fours, hands under the shoulders, feet and knees hip-width apart. Lift each hand in turn and place the heel of the hand where the fingertips were, to reposition your hands one hands-length forward, as shown. Tuck the toes under.

2 On an out-breath, come up on your toes and lift your hips up and back. Keeping your knees bent, push your hands against the floor to send your weight back toward your feet. Lengthen through the spine.

TAKE CARE
If you have back problems, keep the knees bent throughout or do the Alternative (right).

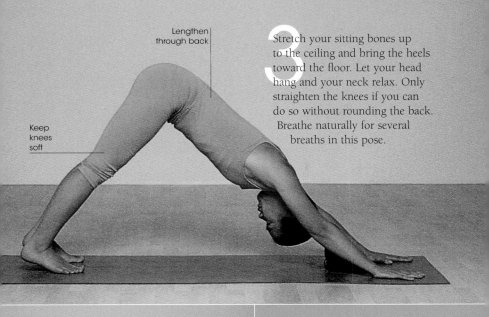

Lengthen
through back

Keep
knees
soft

3 Stretch your sitting bones up to the ceiling and bring the heels toward the floor. Let your head hang and your neck relax. Only straighten the knees if you can do so without rounding the back. Breathe naturally for several breaths in this pose.

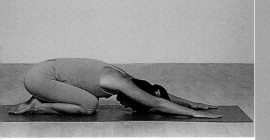

4 On an out-breath, lower the knees to the floor and, keeping your hands still, sit back on your heels in Hare (see p.85). Relax the arms and stay for a few breaths. Feel the stretch through the spine.

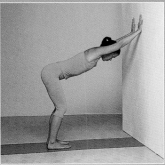

ALTERNATIVE

If you have HBP, a detached retina, or glaucoma, do the pose with your hands against a wall or on a chair.

cobra

Cobra extends the spine, strengthening the muscles in the back and stretching the front of the body. It also opens the chest, strengthens the diaphragm, and releases tension in the shoulders.

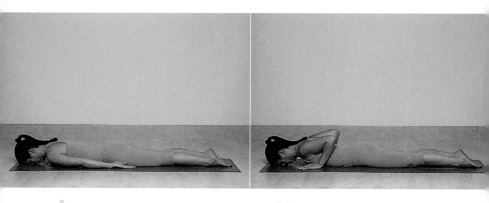

1 Lie on your front, forehead on the floor and feet hip-width apart. Let your arms lie down by your sides, palms facing up. Stretch the feet away along the floor.

2 Place your hands under the shoulders and spread your fingers, middle finger pointing forward. Keep the elbows close to the body and tuck your tailbone under. Roll the shoulders back.

TAKE CARE
- Avoid if you have facet joint problems in the spine.
- If you have arthritis in the neck, keep the head in line with the spine.

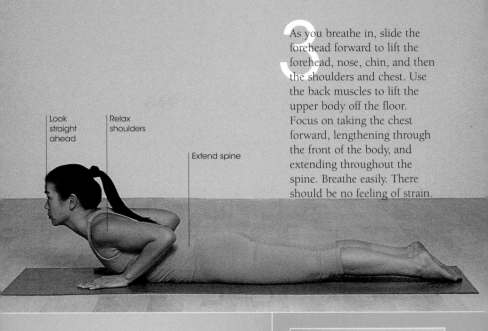

3 As you breathe in, slide the forehead forward to lift the forehead, nose, chin, and then the shoulders and chest. Use the back muscles to lift the upper body off the floor. Focus on taking the chest forward, lengthening through the front of the body, and extending throughout the spine. Breathe easily. There should be no feeling of strain.

Look straight ahead

Relax shoulders

Extend spine

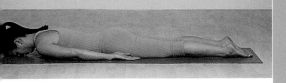

4 Repeat the pose once or twice, resting in between with your forehead on the floor and your arms beside you, palms facing up. Then rest with the head turned to one side.

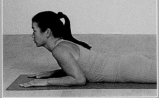

ALTERNATIVE

If you are stiff in the shoulders or have a rounded upper spine (kyphosis), you may prefer to place your hands beside your face and keep your forearms on the floor as you lift up the upper body.

locust

This back-arching posture stretches the whole body and raises the spirits. It provides a balanced strengthening of the back muscles. Practice with the breath to avoid strain and keep the mind focused.

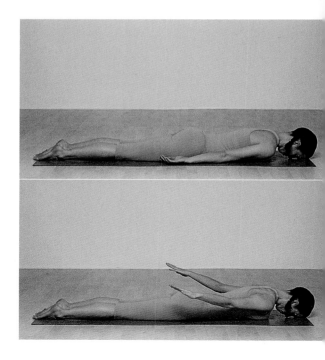

1 Lie on your front with your forehead on the floor, your feet a little apart, and your arms by your sides. Relax completely for a few breaths.

2 Breathing out, stretch the feet away from you along the floor. Stretch the arms up and back behind you like wings. Keep your forehead pressed on the floor.

3 As you breathe in, slide the nose and chin along the floor. Lift the head and the upper body a little. Lift both legs straight up from the hip, contracting the lower back muscles. Feel the whole body lengthening. As you breathe out, slowly lower the body to the floor and relax briefly. Repeat four to six times.

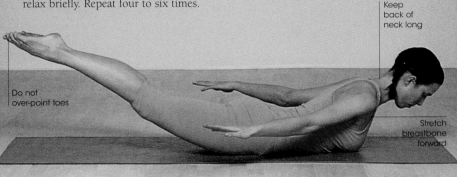

Keep back of neck long

Do not over-point toes

Stretch breastbone forward

4 On the final lowering of the body, turn the head to one side and relax the body completely. Be aware of the lower back rising and falling with the breath.

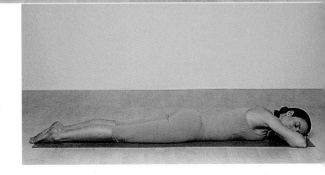

TAKE CARE
Avoid this pose if you have a peptic ulcer, hernia, or spinal facet joint problems.

half bow

The Half Bow posture works the back, while gently stretching the front thigh and hip-flexor muscles. It is a good forerunner to the full Bow and has an invigorating, energizing effect.

1 Lie on your front with your forehead on the floor, your feet a little apart, and your arms by your sides, palms facing up.

2 As you breathe in, stretch your right arm above your head, palm facing the floor. Point the fingers away from the body. Keep resting your forehead on the floor.

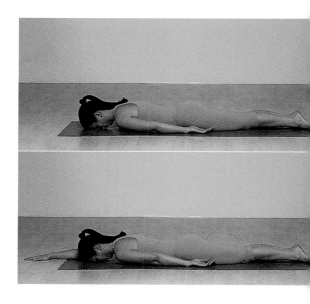

TAKE CARE
- If you have HBP, heart disease, or a hernia, do not hold final position.
- If you have back problems, stop if symptoms are provoked.

Exhaling, bend your left leg so that your calf touches your thigh, and take hold of the front of the ankle with your left hand. Continue to keep your forehead on the floor.

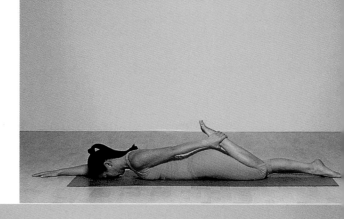

As you breathe in, lift the left thigh, and raise the foot away from the buttock. At the same time, lift the right arm, chest, and head together. Pause as you breathe out. Hold the position for as long as is comfortable, breathing deeply. Then, exhaling, relax the leg and lower yourself back to the floor. Repeat on the other side.

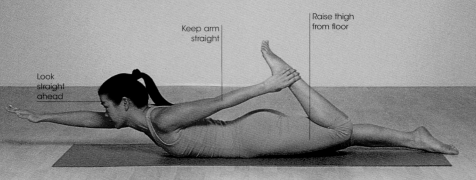

Raise thigh from floor

Keep arm straight

Look straight ahead

bow

Bow strengthens and tones the back and abdominal muscles, and extends the spine. It also opens the chest, stimulating deep breathing, and results in an increased sense of wellbeing.

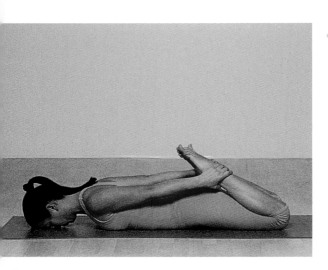

1 Lie on your front, with your legs and feet together, and your arms by your sides, palms facing up. Rest your forehead on the floor. As you breathe out, bend both legs so that the calves touch the thighs. At the same time, reach back with your arms and take hold of the fronts of the ankles.

TAKE CARE
Avoid if you have heart problems, HBP, a hernia, or back problems; start with Half Bow (see p.62).

2 As you breathe in, raise the feet away from the buttocks, and, keeping the arms straight, roll the shoulders back, lifting the thighs, chest, and head together. Pause as you breathe out. Breathing in, raise the feet again, and lift a little higher. Hold the position for as long as is comfortable, breathing deeply.

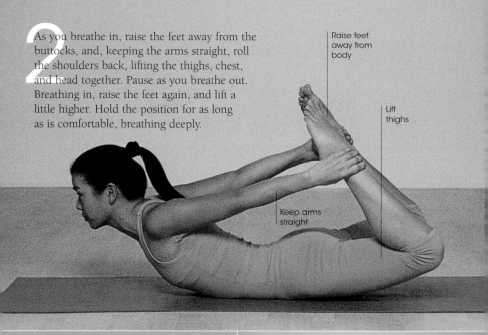

Raise feet away from body

Lift thighs

Keep arms straight

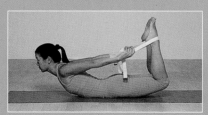

ALTERNATIVE

If you cannot reach your ankles with your hands without straining, use a belt. Wrap it around the ankles and hold the ends with both hands. Draw your chest up as you lift your thighs and raise your feet.

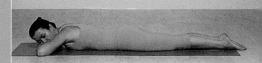

3 On an out-breath, relax the legs and lower your body to the floor. Fold your arms and rest for a few breaths with your head turned to one side, resting on the backs of your hands.

sun
salute

This dynamic sequence energizes the whole body. Try to make the sequence flowing by coordinating movement with breath. After completing the sequence, repeat on the other side of the body.

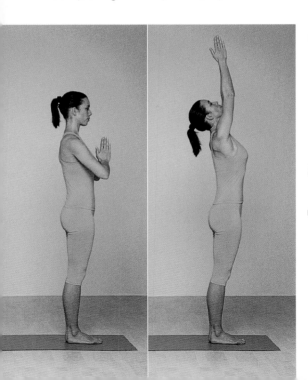

1 Stand up straight with your feet together and your palms pressed together in prayer position in front of your chest. Look straight ahead. Center yourself and then inhale fully.

2 As you breathe in, take your arms out to the sides of your body, turning the palms out, and lift both arms up above your head. Bring your palms together and lift up the breastbone. Open your chest as you look up at your hands. Do not let the head fall back and keep the shoulders relaxed.

Breathing out, fold forward from the hips over bent legs into a relaxed Forward Bend (see p.48). Bend your arms above your head and hold at the elbows. Let the torso hang. Stay in this position for three to four breaths.

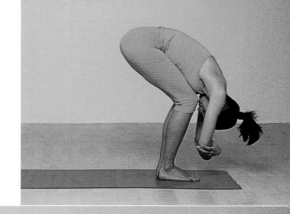

Exhaling, come into Lunge Warrior (see p.54). Take a large step back with your right foot, landing on the ball of the right foot. Lower the right knee to the floor and rest your upper torso on your left thigh. Steeple your fingers. Stretch the breastbone forward and look straight ahead. Stay in the position for three to four breaths. ▶

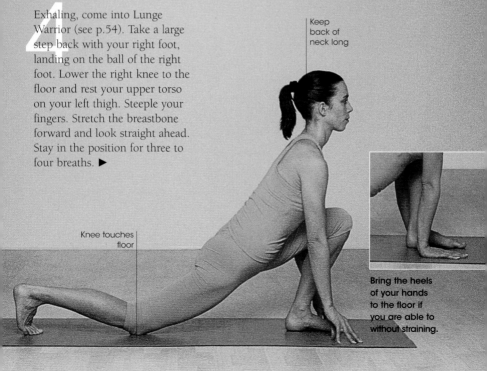

Keep back of neck long

Knee touches floor

Bring the heels of your hands to the floor if you are able to without straining.

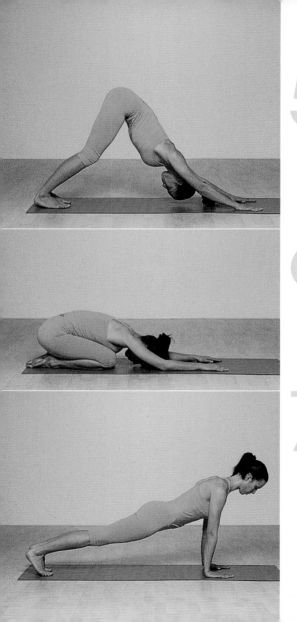

5 Exhale as you step the left foot back to come into Downward Dog (see p.56). Press your heels toward the floor and bend the knees if necessary. Do not force your heels onto the floor. Let your head hang, your neck relax. Stay in the pose for three to four breaths.

6 On an out-breath, bring your knees to the floor, and keeping your hands still, move into Hare (see p.85). Rest in this pose for three to four breaths.

7 Breathing in, bring your body forward and lift your legs and torso off the floor, tucking your toes under. Your hands should be directly beneath your shoulders. Maintain a straight line with your body and legs. Look down at the floor. Hold the position and breathe out.

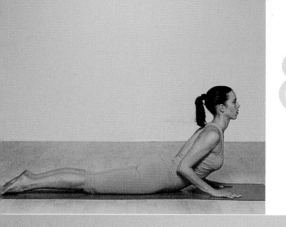

Breathing in, lower yourself to the floor into Cobra (see p.58). Keep the hands directly underneath the shoulders and the elbows tucked in. Focus on taking the chest forward, lengthening through the front of the body, and extending throughout the spine.

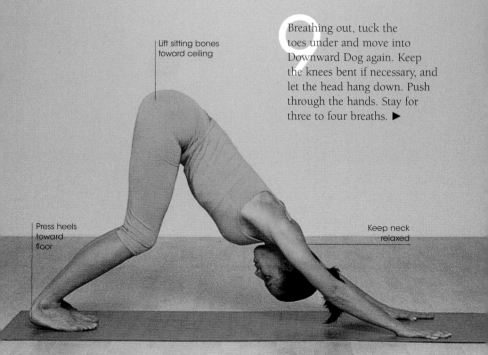

Breathing out, tuck the toes under and move into Downward Dog again. Keep the knees bent if necessary, and let the head hang down. Push through the hands. Stay for three to four breaths. ▶

Lift sitting bones toward ceiling

Press heels toward floor

Keep neck relaxed

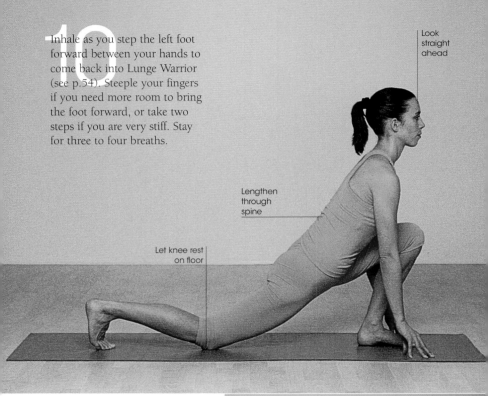

10 Inhale as you step the left foot forward between your hands to come back into Lunge Warrior (see p.54). Steeple your fingers if you need more room to bring the foot forward, or take two steps if you are very stiff. Stay for three to four breaths.

Look straight ahead

Lengthen through spine

Let knee rest on floor

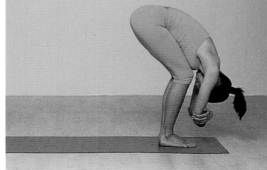

11 As you exhale, bring your right foot forward to join the left foot and come into an easy Forward Bend with bent legs (see p.48). Bend your arms above your head and hold onto the elbows. Relax in this position for three to four breaths.

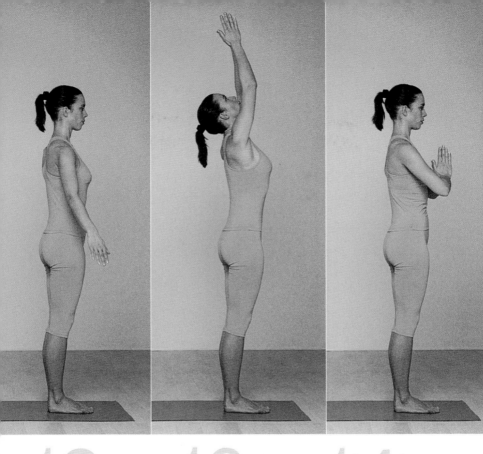

Breathing in, roll the body up slowly, keeping the knees bent until you are completely upright. Breathe out once when you are standing up straight.

Breathing in, circle your arms out to the sides and then over your head. Bring the palms together and look up at your hands. Lift the breastbone, but do not bend backward.

Breathing out, bring your arms down in front of your chest in prayer position. Look straight ahead and breathe easily for a few minutes. Repeat the sequence on the other side.

bridge

Bridge is a back-arching posture that also opens the chest and releases neck and shoulder tension. It is especially soothing if practiced moving on the out-breath only.

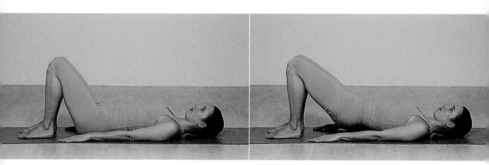

1 Lie on your back with your knees pulled up and your feet hip-width apart. Allow a hand's length of space between the hips and the heels. Have the arms alongside the body with the palms facing down. Draw the chin a little down toward the chest, to lengthen the back of the neck.

2 Breathe in, feeling the length of your back on the floor. As you breathe out, push your feet against the floor to lift the hips and then the back off the floor as far as you comfortably can. Make sure your feet are directly beneath the knees, especially if you have knee problems.

TAKE CARE
If you have neck problems, make sure the back of the neck stays long throughout.

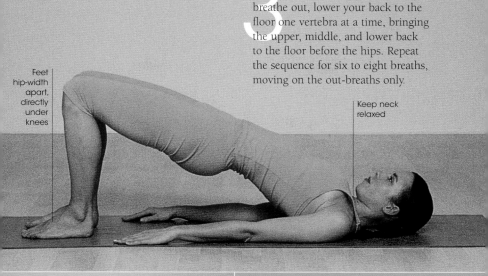

3 Hold the pose and breathe in. As you breathe out, lower your back to the floor one vertebra at a time, bringing the upper, middle, and lower back to the floor before the hips. Repeat the sequence for six to eight breaths, moving on the out-breaths only.

Feet hip-width apart, directly under knees

Keep neck relaxed

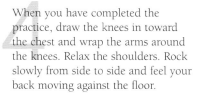

4 When you have completed the practice, draw the knees in toward the chest and wrap the arms around the knees. Relax the shoulders. Rock slowly from side to side and feel your back moving against the floor.

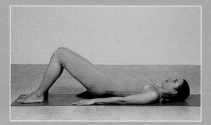

ALTERNATIVE

If you have a back problem, try taking the feet a little farther away from the hips when you begin, and lift only the hips off the floor, not the whole back.

legs
up the wall

Inverted postures can be particularly restorative, and you do not need to be able to do a Headstand to reap the benefits of inversion. Try Legs up the Wall first if you are new to inverted postures.

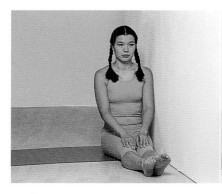
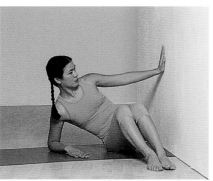

1 Sit up straight with your left hip against a wall. Place your hands on your thighs and breathe easily for a few moments. Draw the knees up.

2 Lean over on to your right elbow and place the left hand against the wall. Swivel your trunk through 90 degrees so that your legs are against the wall and your hips close to the base of it.

TAKE CARE
• If you have HBP, Legs up the Wall is the only suitable inverted posture.
• If you have LBP, come out of any inverted postures really slowly.

3 Bend your elbows and bring your hands to rest on your stomach. Relax the legs up the wall and stay quietly in this position, observing the flow of the natural breath for two to three minutes.

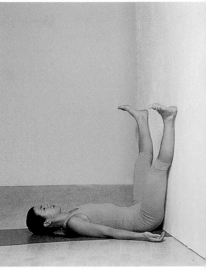

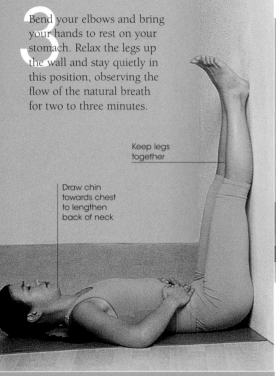

Keep legs together

Draw chin towards chest to lengthen back of neck

4 Separate the feet, and let your arms rest by your sides, palms up, for a few breaths. To come out of the pose, draw the knees over the chest and roll over to one side. Stay in this position for a few breaths before sitting up. Once sitting, wait for a few breaths before standing up.

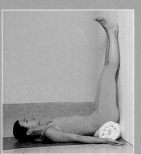

ALTERNATIVE
Place a soft bolster or cushion under the hips if your back is not comfortable when flat on the floor.

half shoulder stand

This gentle version of Shoulder Stand is restorative, quietening the mind while resting the legs and lower body. By using a wall for support, it is easy to learn how to do this inversion.

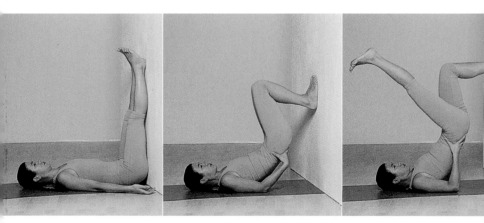

1 Sit with your left hip against a wall. Move into Legs up the Wall (see p.74).

2 Place the feet against the wall and push, raising the hips. Bring the hands to the backs of the hipbones.

3 Lift the heels from the wall and raise the hips higher. Take the right foot off the wall and bring over your head.

TAKE CARE
If you have HBP, a heart condition, a detached retina, glaucoma, neck problems, or are overweight, do Legs up the Wall (see p.74).

Take the left foot off the wall. Relax the neck and stay for several breaths. Pull the chin gently toward the chest to lengthen the back of the neck. Breathe normally, stretching the soles of the feet toward the ceiling and lengthening through the legs and spine.

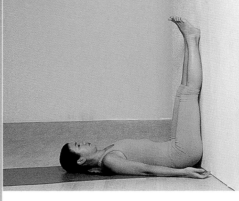

Keep legs
straight and
together

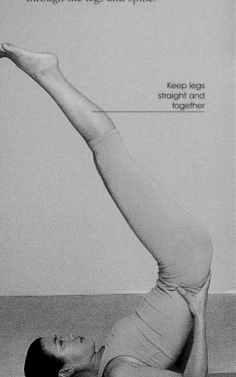

Bend your right knee to bring the sole of your right foot back to the wall. Then bring your left foot to the wall. Lower your spine to the floor, keeping the back supported as you come down. Take your arms out to the side.

To come out of the pose, draw the knees over the chest and roll onto your right side. Stay with the head down for several breaths. Sit up slowly, particularly if you have LBP.

Keep elbows well tucked
in for support

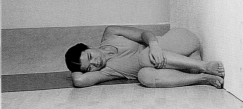

easy fish

This posture opens the hips and shoulders, while supporting the back.
Easy Fish provides an excellent counterstretch for the back and the
neck after doing the Half Shoulder Stand (see p.76).

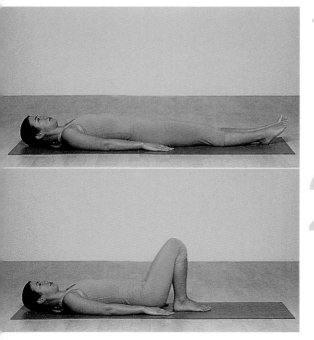

1 Lie on your back with your
legs outstretched and your
feet hip-width apart. Place
your arms by your sides,
palms facing down. Look
up at the ceiling.

2 Pull up the knees and place
the soles of your feet flat
on the floor close to the
hips. Lengthen the back
of the neck by drawing the
chin down a little toward
the chest.

3 Cross your feet at the ankles, and allow the knees to drop out to the sides – right knee to the right side, left knee to the left – so that you are lying in a cross-legged position. Let the hip joints relax and open. Do not overarch the back.

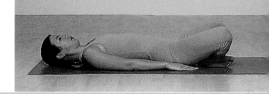

4 Bring your arms up and clasp your hands to cradle the head. Let the elbows sink to the floor. Observe the natural rise and fall of the abdomen with the breath for several breaths. Uncross the ankles, cross them the other way, and stay for several more breaths. To come out of the pose, bring the knees back together and slide the feet away.

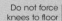

Do not force knees to floor

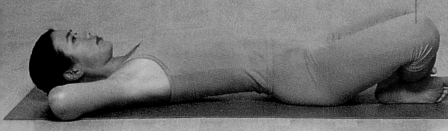

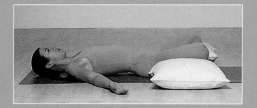

ALTERNATIVE

If you have lower back pain, sacroiliac problems, or simply stiff hips, support either or both legs by tucking a bolster or pillow under the thighs. Then let the thighs relax down onto the support.

roaring
lion

Roaring Lion posture is a great stress reliever. It stretches the face, jaw, and throat, while simultaneously releasing any sense of being under pressure, whether from the demands of work or home.

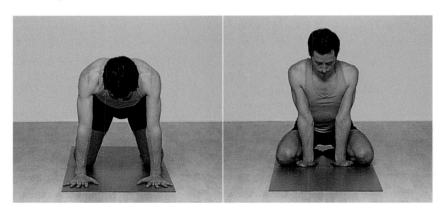

1 Begin on all fours, the hands directly under the shoulders, the feet and knees about hip-width apart. Spread your fingers and look down.

2 Sit back on your heels with the knees wider than the hips and the feet close together. Position the hands on the floor inside the knees, and turn the hands so that the heels of the hands point forward. Lift the breastbone and look slightly forward.

Breathe in deeply. As you breathe out, open your mouth wide and stretch the tip of the tongue down to the chin. Open the eyes wide and look up, as you exhale with a soft, continuous "haaaa" sound. The sound should be soft, not harsh or unduly loud, and should last the length of the exhalation. If your throat feels rough afterward, you are practicing too strongly.

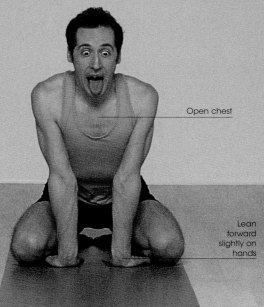

Open chest

Lean forward slightly on hands

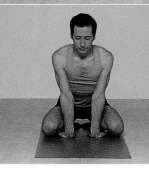

As you breathe in, slowly pull in the relaxed tongue, relax the face, and close the mouth. Breathe normally for a few breaths, feeling the effects, then repeat two or three times.

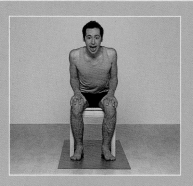

ALTERNATIVE

If you have knee problems or painful wrists, sit on a chair. Lean forward, the hands placed lightly on the thighs.

cat

Cat is practiced slowly, with the movements initiated from the tailbone. It works the back, easing out tension and strengthening the muscles. Learn the positions first, then link them to the breath.

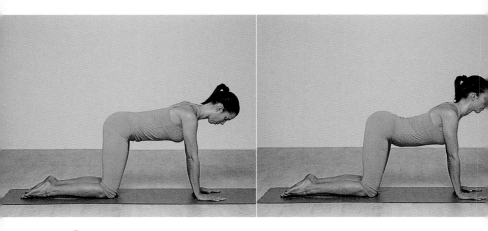

1 Kneel on all fours, hands under the shoulders and knees under the hips. Push the hands into the floor to prevent the shoulders from sagging. Look down at the floor.

2 As you breathe in, begin to lift the tailbone up away from the floor, so that the lower back dips toward the floor. Continue to lift the tailbone and feel first the middle of the back dip, then the upper back. Look at the floor about 3 ft (1 m) in front of you.

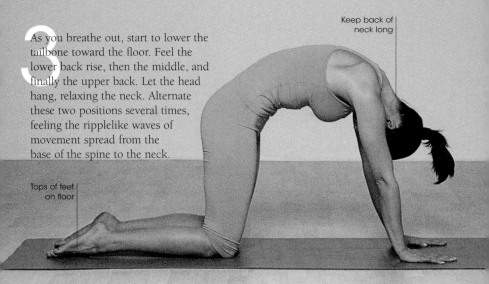

3 As you breathe out, start to lower the tailbone toward the floor. Feel the lower back rise, then the middle, and finally the upper back. Let the head hang, relaxing the neck. Alternate these two positions several times, feeling the ripplelike waves of movement spread from the base of the spine to the neck.

Keep back of neck long

Tops of feet on floor

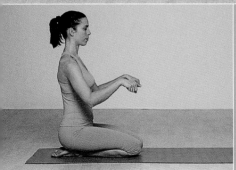

4 On an out-breath, sit back on your heels with your arms in front. Slowly circle the hands at the wrists a few times in each direction to ease them after this weight-bearing posture.

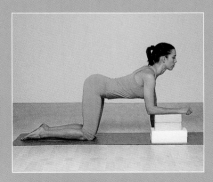

ALTERNATIVE

If one or both your wrists are painful when your hands are bearing your weight or if you have weak wrists, support the body by placing one or both forearms on blocks.

cat
balance

This variation of the Cat pose is unusual in that it stretches the body diagonally. It also encourages balance and a sense of focus. Keep the spine and pelvis in a neutral position throughout.

1 Kneel on all fours, the knees beneath the hips, the feet and knees a little apart. Look down at the floor. Spread the fingers and hold the neck in line.

2 On an in-breath, lift the left leg and stretch it out behind you. Do not look up as this tightens the neck. Pause for a few breaths to get your balance.

3 On an in-breath, slowly take the right arm out in front, parallel to the floor. Stretch the raised hand and foot away from each other. Breathe easily. Slowly release the pose and repeat, stretching out the right leg and the left arm.

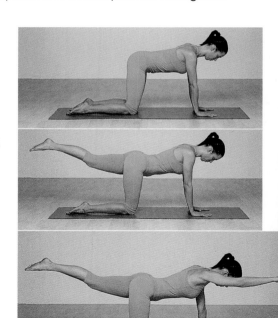

hare

Hare gently stretches the back, hips, knees, and ankles. It is a restorative pose that helps you develop a deep sense of calm by taking your attention inward. (For alternatives, see Child, p.87.)

1 Kneel and sit back on your heels, looking straight ahead. Bring the breastbone up and relax the shoulders. Let your arms hang on each side of the body. Lengthen through the spine. Breathe in.

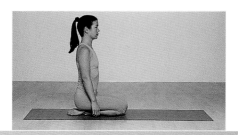

2 As you exhale, fold forward from the hips, stretching the arms out along the floor in front of you and bringing the forehead to the floor between the arms. Stay for several breaths. To come out of the pose, walk your hands toward your body and sit up on your heels.

If your ankles are uncomfortable, place a folded cloth beneath them for support.

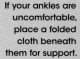

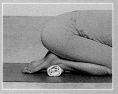

Hands and elbows flat on floor

child

Child is a deeply calming pose that gently stretches the spine and postural muscles in the back, while taking your attention inward. It is a good posture for developing breath awareness.

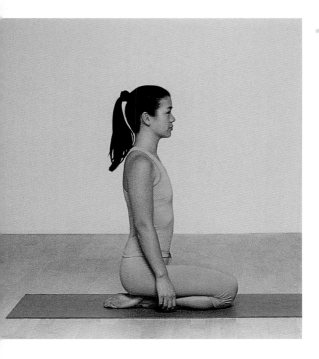

1 Kneel and sit back on your heels. Keep the breastbone up and the shoulders relaxed. Allow your arms to hang down on each side of your body. Lengthen through the spine and look straight ahead. Breathe in.

2 As you exhale, fold forward, tucking the chin in to bring the head to the floor. Let the weight of the arms pull the shoulders gently toward the floor. Stay for several breaths. To come out of the pose, bring the palms of your hands to the floor and push up slowly.

Feel stretch across upper back

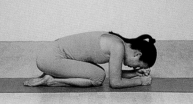

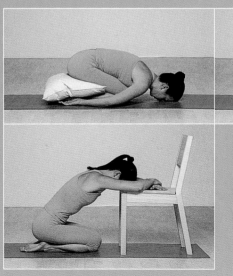

ALTERNATIVES

If your knees are uncomfortable, place a small pillow between the hips and the heels to lift the hips a little. If you find it difficult to bring your head to the floor, rest it on your two fists, one on top of the other. If you have HBP, a detached retina, glaucoma, or back problems, rest your head on the seat of a chair.

seated
forward stretch

This posture has marked quietening effects and is often used in yoga therapy to reduce stress. It encourages flexibility in the spine and hamstrings, and allows you to focus on inner awareness.

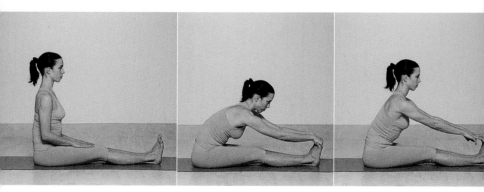

1 Set a firm pillow or bolster close by. Sit with your legs straight out in front of you, feet together. Let your hands rest lightly on your thighs. Look straight ahead and take a few breaths to center yourself.

2 Breathing out, lift the breastbone and lengthen the spine. Relax the shoulders. Stretch forward from the hips and hold the toes, ankles, or shins, depending on your level of flexibility.

3 As you breathe in, lift up the breastbone and lengthen the spine, keeping hold of the toes. Keep the legs and arms straight, and look straight ahead.

4 As you breathe out, fold forward again, bending the elbows and relaxing the neck. Bring your head to your knees, rounding your back. Keep the legs straight. Repeat Steps 3 and 4 for four to six breaths.

Keep neck relaxed

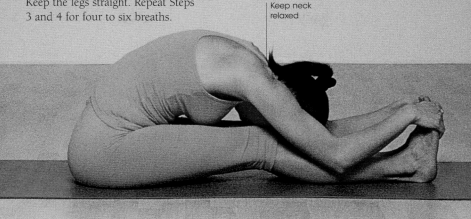

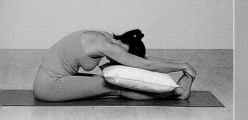

5 Place a firm pillow, bolster, or folded blanket on your legs below your knees. Relax forward over the support and hold for a farther four to six breaths. Be aware of the flow of the natural breath.

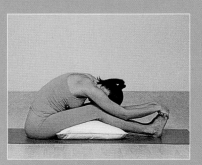

ALTERNATIVE

If you have back problems, a hernia, or tight hamstrings, do not strain to reach toes. Place a pillow under the knees.

cobbler

Cobbler pose opens the hips, while lengthening the spine upward. Practiced with the breath, it is one of the most quietening of all yoga postures, and a wonderful stress reliever.

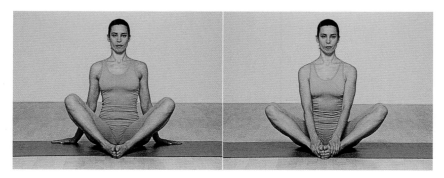

1 Sit with your legs stretched out in front of you. Place your hands on the floor on either side of your body and lean back a little. Bend the knees and swing the soles of your feet together on the floor in front of you.

2 Reach forward and clasp the hands around the feet. Breathing in, sit up straight, lifting the breastbone and lengthening the spine upward. Look straight ahead.

TAKE CARE
• If your back rounds, sit on a foam block or small cushion.
• If you have stiff hips, place a pillow under each thigh for support.

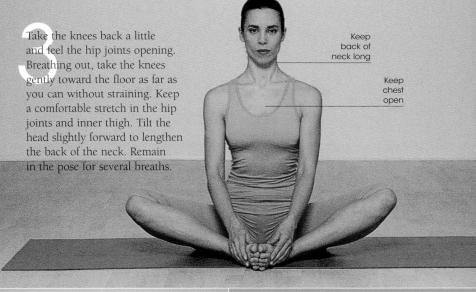

3 Take the knees back a little and feel the hip joints opening. Breathing out, take the knees gently toward the floor as far as you can without straining. Keep a comfortable stretch in the hip joints and inner thigh. Tilt the head slightly forward to lengthen the back of the neck. Remain in the pose for several breaths.

Keep back of neck long

Keep chest open

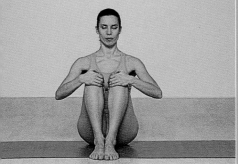

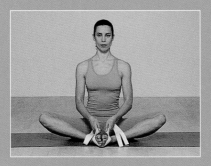

4 To come out of the pose, release the feet and pull the knees together. Place your hands on your knees and roll the legs from side to side several times to ease the hips.

ALTERNATIVE

If you find it difficult to sit up straight while holding onto the feet, use a belt looped around the feet. Hold onto the belt near to the feet, so the shoulders are gently pulled down.

kneeling
stretch sequence

This is a calming sequence that helps you unwind and balance your energy. It is especially beneficial at the end of a stressful day, when it will refresh your mind and body, enabling you to enjoy the evening.

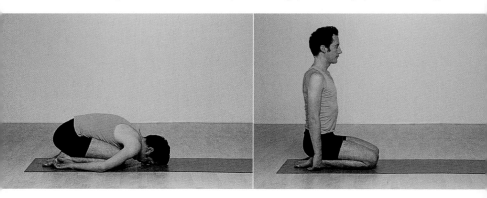

1 Kneel and sit back on your heels, your arms by the sides of your body. As you breathe out, fold forward into Child (see p.86), bringing the upper body onto the thighs.

2 Breathe in and come back up to sitting on your heels. Let your arms hang down by the sides of your body. Look straight ahead. Breathe out.

TAKE CARE
• Take your time to learn the sequence, matching it to the breathing pattern.
• Practice within your natural breathing capacity, gradually developing slow, rhythmic breathing.

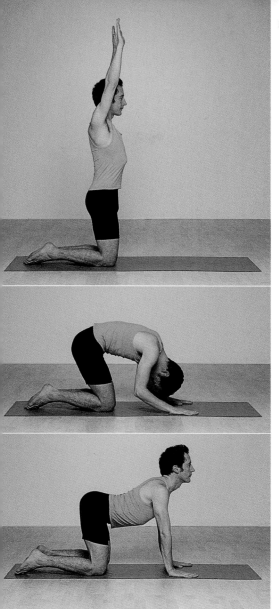

Breathing in, come up onto your knees. At the same time, raise the arms up above the head. Soften the elbows as the arms come up, palms facing forward, shoulders relaxed. Look straight ahead.

Breathing out, curl the tailbone under and bring the hips down toward the heels, stopping before you reach them. Let the hands come lightly to the floor in front of you and the head hang in a kneeling Forward Bend.

Breathing in, bring the head and chest up, so that you are in an all-fours position. Stretch the breastbone forward and bring the tailbone up, letting the back sink down into the first part of Cat (see p.82). ▶

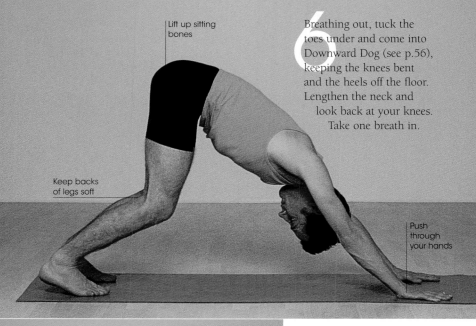

Lift up sitting
bones

Keep backs
of legs soft

6 Breathing out, tuck the
toes under and come into
Downward Dog (see p.56),
keeping the knees bent
and the heels off the floor.
Lengthen the neck and
look back at your knees.
Take one breath in.

Push
through
your hands

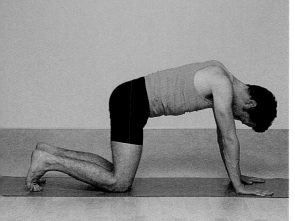

7 Breathing out, come back
onto all fours, your knees
directly underneath your
hips. Look down at the
floor. Breathe in.

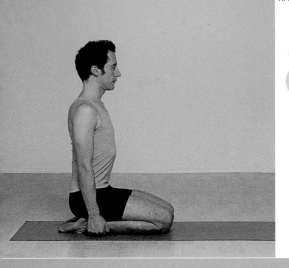

8 Breathing out, come back up to kneeling, sitting on your heels. Let your arms hang down by your sides. Look straight ahead and take a breath in.

9 Breathing out, fold forward from the hips, bringing your forehead to the floor. Slide the hands forward beyond your head into Hare (see p.85). Rest in this pose for several breaths, then push up slowly with your hands. Repeat the entire sequence twice more.

Feel stretch across back

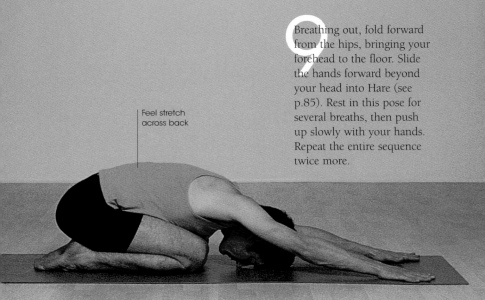

sitting
twist

Sitting twists help to maintain flexibility in the back while easing out muscle tension. This posture is also very stress-relieving because it helps you connect with your breath at a deep level.

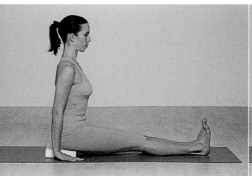 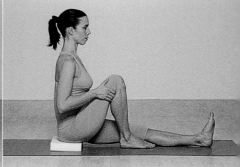

1 Sit on a foam block or small cushion, with the legs straight out in front of you and the feet together. Lift the breastbone and lengthen the spine upward. Relax the shoulders and look straight ahead.

2 Place your hands under the right knee and pull the knee up. Flex the left foot and stretch the heel of the left leg away from you. Continue to look straight ahead.

TAKE CARE
Twist within comfortable limits. It is important to turn the neck last, avoiding any sense of strain in this area.

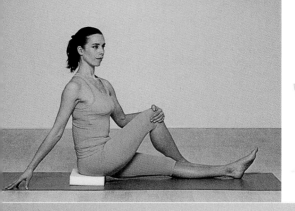

Take the right foot across the left leg, setting it down beside the left calf. Clasp both hands over the bent knee and lengthen the spine. Bring the fingers of the right hand to the floor behind you. Breathe in as you lengthen through the upper body.

Breathing out, turn your abdomen, waist, ribcage, shoulders, and finally the head to the right as far as you comfortably can. As you turn, straighten the left arm, setting it against the outside of the bent knee, fingers stretched. Stay in the posture for four to six breaths, then slowly and smoothly release the twist, return to the starting position, and repeat on the other side.

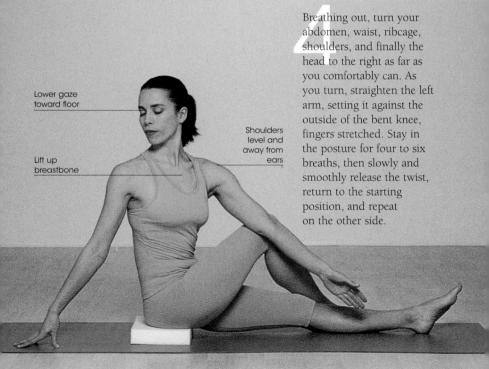

Lower gaze toward floor

Lift up breastbone

Shoulders level and away from ears

chair
twist

Tension in the neck, shoulders, and lower back may set in toward the end of the day after spending hours at your desk. Break up the day and release the tension by doing the Chair Twist in your office.

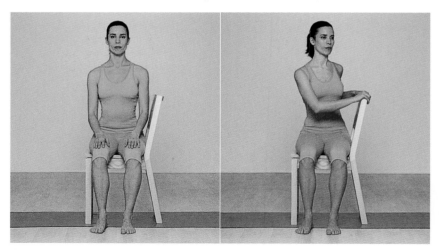

1 Sit sideways on the chair, with your feet on the ground. If the chair is too high, place a telephone directory or similar book under your feet. Place your hands on your thighs and look straight ahead.

2 Lift up the breastbone and take hold of the back of the chair with both hands. Relax the shoulders. Look down slightly. Breathing out, begin to turn the upper body toward the back of the chair, starting with the stomach.

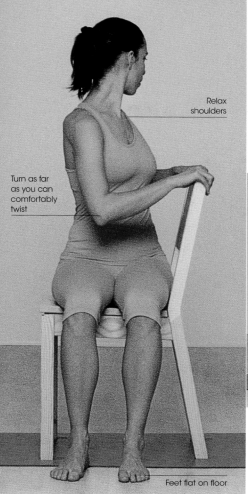

Relax
shoulders

Turn as far
as you can
comfortably
twist

Feet flat on floor

Still breathing out, turn the waist,
rib cage, and shoulders, keeping
the breastbone up and shoulders
relaxed. Finally, turn the head as
far as it will comfortably go. Relax
the face and connect with the
breath for several breaths.

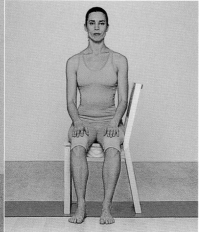

On an out-breath, slowly release
the pose and come back to the
starting position. Swivel around
on the chair to face the opposite
direction and practice the posture
on the other side.

TAKE CARE
Turn each part of the trunk only to your maximum
comfortable limit: there should be no strain at any time.

breathing
practices & mudras

Breathing practices improve your awareness of the breath and are particularly useful in quietening the mind for meditation. Mudras are traditional hand gestures that help you to center yourself.

The breathing practices described on these four pages will help improve your breath awareness and encourage calmness and mental clarity. They are generally practiced after doing some yoga postures, or some simple stretching. Physical movement helps loosen up the body, so that it is easier for you to be relaxed during the breathing practices. You might like to use a mudra in conjunction with a breathing practice to improve its effectiveness.

Audible breath

A simple but effective breathing practice to begin with is known as audible breath. This practice helps to make the breath smooth and even, calms and centers the mind, and is

a proven stress reliever. It can also be used during posture work to help you to remain focused.

Begin with the preliminary practice described below. When you have gotten a feel for this, try to

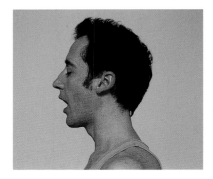

Breathe through the mouth. Slightly close the throat and make a sighing "Ahhhh" sound as you breathe in and a sighing "Haaa" sound as you breathe out.

achieve the same sound in the throat while breathing with your mouth closed. It helps to think that you are breathing through a hole in the front of the throat. Breathe smoothly and evenly, and keep your awareness on the breath. The sound of the breath can be subtle; only you need hear it.

Using mudras

There are many mudras, or hand gestures, used in yoga practice. The centering mudra shown on this page (see right) helps you to quieten quickly when you are feeling stressed. This enables you to break the stress cycle effortlessly, making you feel much calmer within minutes. Practicing this mudra also acts to remind you of the link between the individual and universal consciousness – that we are all interconnected, never unsupported.

The centering mudra can be very helpful at any time of the day, whatever your situation. It can be used in an unobtrusive way at work, socially, and at times of stress, with the hands in any convenient position – they do not have to be supported.

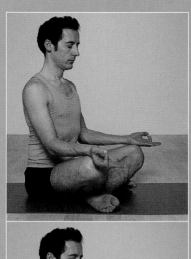

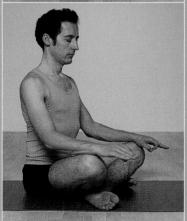

MUDRA FOR CENTERING

Bring the tip of each index finger and thumb together lightly. Rest the hands on the thighs or the knees. During the day, have the palms facing up, and after dark have them facing down.

alternate nostril breathing

Breathing through alternate nostrils has a balancing effect on the mind, body, and emotions. As you practice the breathing, let go of any tension in the body. If you are left-handed, adapt the instructions below to suit. Do several rounds. When you are comfortable with the practice, begin to lengthen the out-breath until it is twice as long as the in-breath.

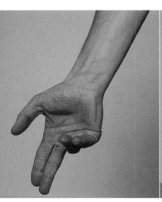 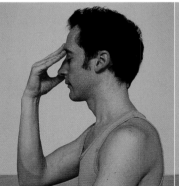 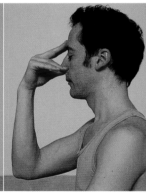

1 Sit cross-legged on the floor. Lift the breastbone and relax the shoulders. Take your right hand and separate the index and middle fingers from the thumb and the ring and little finger. Place the index and middle fingers in the center of the forehead.

2 Connect with your natural breath. Close the right nostril with your thumb and breathe in through the left nostril.

3 Close the left nostril with your ring and little finger and open the right. Breathe out through the right, then breathe back in through the right. Close the right nostril, open the left, and breathe out through that. This completes one round.

sounds breathing

This practice uses the vibrational power of sound to relax the body and mind, and helps to make the breath smooth and even. Once you are familiar with the practice, you can do it without making a sound. Inhale, and as you exhale soundlessly, simply visualize the "ahhhh," "ohhhh," and "mmmm" sounds for the length of each out-breath.

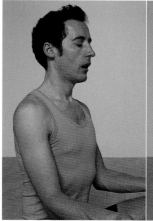 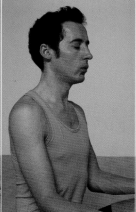 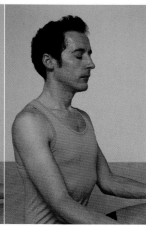

1 Sit cross-legged and close your eyes. Lift the breastbone and relax the shoulders. Inhale and, as you breathe out, make the sound "ahhhh." Feel the vibrations in the abdomen. Repeat twice more.

2 Breathe in and, as you breathe out, make the sound "ohhhh" for the length of the out-breath. This time, feel the vibrations in the chest. Repeat this sound twice more.

3 For the length of the next out-breath, make the sound "mmmm." As you do so, feel the vibrations in the throat and the head. Repeat this sound twice more. Be aware of the stillness within, then open your eyes.

meditation

Meditation is a practice that allows the mind to quieten, giving a lasting sense of inner peace and harmony. It helps keep your mind clear throughout the day and can aid sleep at night.

Sit in a comfortable but alert way, either cross-legged on the floor (using a block, pillow, or blanket if you prefer) or upright in a chair. Bring the index finger and thumb of each hand together and rest the hands on your knees or thighs. This is the mudra that allows you to center yourself more effectively and connects you to the universal consciousness (see p.101).

PRACTICAL MATTERS

• Choose a posture that you will be able to sustain easily for some time; for example, sitting cross-legged, kneeling, or sitting upright on a chair.
• Make sure the temperature of the room is comfortable. You may need to put on some warmer clothes if you have been doing posture work.

Scan the body, letting go of any tension you are holding (in your face, neck, shoulders, upper body, hips, legs, and feet). Close your eyes and let your breath settle into an easy, regular rhythm. Do not try actively to shut out any noises or other sensations. Let them exist, and withdraw your senses from them as you focus on your breath. Be aware of the coolness of the air in the openings of the nostrils as you breathe in and the warmth of the air there as you breathe out.

To begin with, thoughts will inevitably arise and sensations will distract you. You cannot force the mind to be empty. But do not let yourself react to these disturbances.

Observe them objectively as they come into the mind and let them go as you continue to focus on the breath. Do not let yourself be carried away on a train of thought.

Using visualization

Bring your awareness to your natural breath. As you draw the breath in, visualize the breath entering your body through the base of your spine and moving gently up the spine until it fills your lungs. As you breathe out, visualize the breath flowing back down the spine and leaving the body.

Visualize the breath as a fine mist or as a soft white light. Alternatively, if you find visualization difficult, simply focus on the sense of movement as the breath passes up and down the spine. You may like to say to yourself "up" as you breathe in, and "down" as you breathe out.

Let the practice be easy, without any sense of strain. If you notice that your mind has wandered, gently bring it back to "seeing" the flow of the breath up and down the spine. After two to three minutes you will

notice that you are feeling quietly energized and calmer than before.

Practice this visualization meditation for up to 10 minutes, then open your eyes. Once you are accustomed to the practice, you will be able to use it in any situation and posture – sitting or standing, eyes open or closed, and the hands relaxed in any comfortable position.

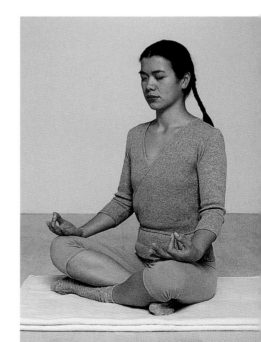

relaxation

Stress affects the mind and the body equally. It can be difficult for a busy mind to quieten directly, but when you learn to relax the body, you will find your mind soon settles and becomes calm.

Relaxation is a skill that improves with regular practice, as the body and mind become accustomed to releasing tension.

There are two relaxation practices described on the next four pages. The instant relaxation practice can be used at any time of the day or night, anywhere, sitting or standing. For the 10-minute relaxation practice, you will need to lie down in a place where you are guaranteed privacy and quiet for at least 10 minutes. It provides a deep relaxation and is ideal when you have plenty of time.

Relaxation benefits

Use the instant relaxation technique (see opposite) whenever you feel stress building up during the day.

Once you have learned this simple and unobtrusive practice, you will also find it extremely useful to try in specific situations, for example, just before a high-pressure meeting, interview, or presentation.

Lying down in deep relaxation for ten minutes or so allows you to recharge your batteries and let go of any feeling of being under pressure. Many people find it especially beneficial to practice deep relaxation at the end of their yoga session, to reinforce the restorative and regenerative benefits. Try to make sure you will not be disturbed. Loosen any tight clothing and wear a sweater or cover yourself with a blanket: the body loses heat as the blood vessels in the skin relax.

instant relaxation

It is invaluable to be able to relax at any time, in any situation. Using this simple technique, you will quickly learn to be composed and stress-free, no matter what is going on around you. Repeat this instant relaxation practice as soon as you begin to feel any tension building up again.

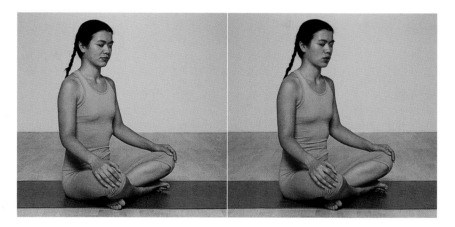

1 Sit cross-legged on the floor, your hands resting on your knees. Close your eyes. Turn your attention inward and become aware of the flow of the natural breath. Breathe in through the nose as you take your awareness to your jaw.

2 Breathe out in an even stream through slightly pursed lips, softly "blowing the breath away" and with it the stress in your jaw. With the next in-breath, be aware of the shoulders, and then blow out the tension with the out-breath. On the next in-breath, focus on the hands. As you breathe out, let them become passive. Move your awareness between these areas for several breaths, keeping each one relaxed and soft.

10-minute relaxation

Try recording this guided relaxation, or ask a friend to read it to you slowly. This allows you to relax to the deepest level. Lie on your back with your legs outstretched, feet more than hip-width apart. Let the feet roll out. (If you have lower back problems, keep your knees bent.) Ease the shoulders down to the floor. Take the arms away from the body and turn the inner elbows and palms up to the ceiling. Lengthen the back of the neck, bringing the chin toward the chest. Close the eyes. Let the body become still.

Scanning the body

Take your awareness around each part of the right side of the body. Be aware of the thumb, fingers, palm of right hand, back of hand, wrist, lower arm, elbow, upper arm, shoulder, armpit, right side of chest, right side of waist, right hip, right thigh, kneecap, back of knee, shin, calf muscle, ankle, heel, sole of foot, top of foot, toes.

Now take your attention to the left side of the body. Be aware of the thumb, fingers, palm of the left hand, back of hand, wrist. Be aware of the lower arm, elbow, upper arm, shoulder, armpit, left side of chest, left side of waist, left hip. Now be aware of the left thigh, kneecap, back of knee, shin, calf muscle, ankle, heel, sole of foot, top of foot, toes.

Take your awareness to the back of the body. Be aware of the back of the head, back of the neck, backs of shoulders, left shoulder blade, right shoulder blade, middle of back, lower back, left buttock, right buttock, back of left thigh, back of right thigh, back of left knee, back of right knee, left calf, right calf, left heel, right heel, sole of left foot, sole of right foot.

Take your attention to the top of your head. Now to the front of the body. Be aware of the forehead, left eyebrow, right eyebrow, space between eyebrows, left eyelid, right eyelid, left eyeball, right eyeball. Be aware of the bridge of the nose, left nostril, right nostril, left cheekbone, right cheekbone, upper lip, inside the mouth – teeth, gums, tongue – the lower lip, chin, under the chin, front of throat, left side of neck, right side of neck, left collarbone, right collarbone, left side of chest, right side of chest, front of chest, abdomen. Now be aware of the whole body.

Focusing inwards

Turn your attention inward and feel how tranquil your body has become. Become aware of the quietness of your breath, which does not disturb the stillness of your body as it flows gently in and out. Stay with your breath for a little while, and as you do, experience the sense of inner quietness, inner peace – feel connected with your inner self at the deepest level. Stay in this relaxing posture for two to 10 minutes.

Coming out

When you are ready, draw your awareness outward again. Be aware of the floor beneath you, the room around you, the sounds that you can hear. Begin to breathe a little more deeply, then start slowly to move the fingers and toes, ankles, arms, and legs. Shrug the shoulders, move the neck, face, and scalp. Take the arms back behind the head and stretch out the body right to the fingertips and down to the heels and toes. Now draw the knees over the chest, wrap the arms around the knees, relax the shoulders, and rock slowly from side to side, feeling your back move against the floor. Now roll over to the right and sit up slowly.

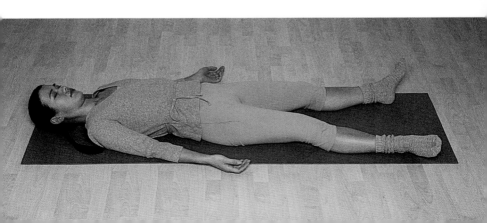

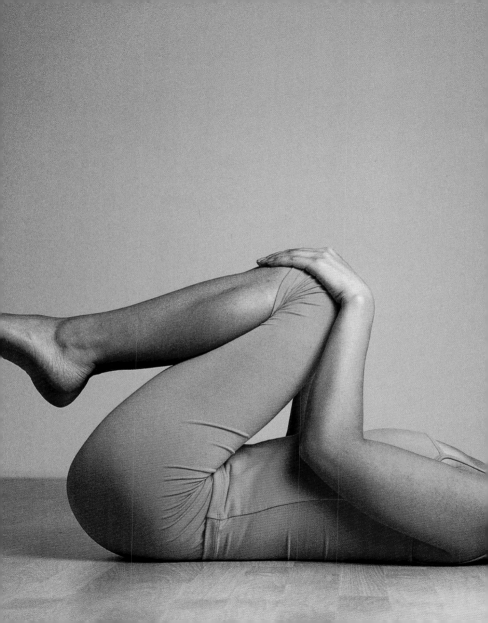

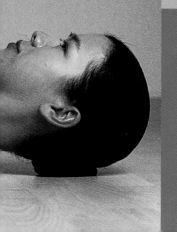

programs

Here are eight programs for those times in the day when you need to de-stress. Remember to take time to center yourself before doing them and time to absorb their effects afterward. Their benefits will be greatly enhanced if you remember that yoga is also about lifestyle and attitude.

1 preparing for the day

Early morning is the traditional time for yoga practice. Take a few moments to become centered first. This will enable you to develop a sense of calm that will help see you through any stresses in the day ahead. You may feel stiff after sleep, so work gently to open up tight areas, letting your energy flow easily around the body.

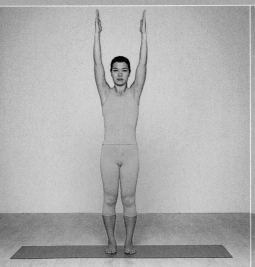

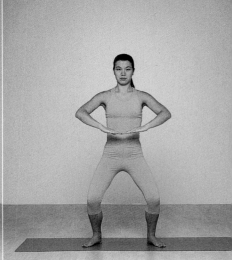

❶ Standing Upward Stretch (see p.38)

❷ French Press Stretch (see p.35)

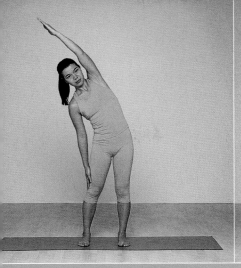

3 Standing Side Stretch (see p.41)

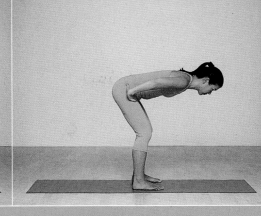

4 Half Forward Bend (see p.39)

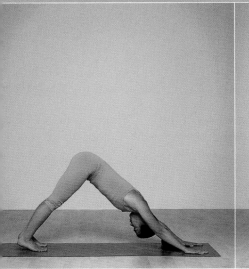

5 Downward Dog (see pp.56–57)

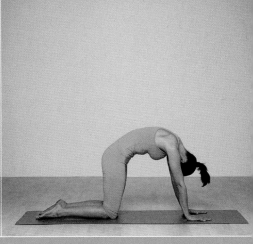

6 Cat (see pp.82–83)

2 work-time
stretch

Working indoors in an office environment can make you feel in need of a good stretch. This program does not require you to get down on the floor; you can stand or sit on an upright chair. The postures may be used together during a short break, but are equally effective practiced separately at intervals during your working hours.

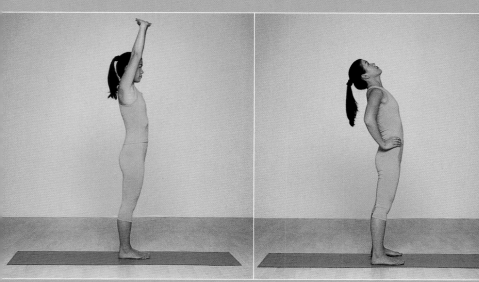

1 Standing Arm Stretches (see p.34)

2 Standing Back Arch (see p.40)

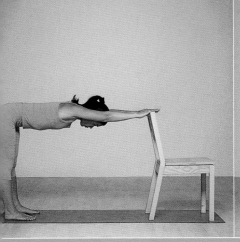

3 Forward Bend using a chair (see p.49)

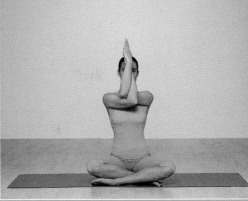

4 Eagle (see pp.44–45)

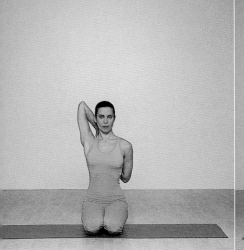

5 Cow (see pp.46–47)

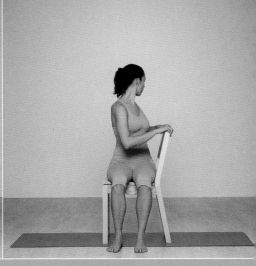

6 Chair Twist (see pp.98–99)

3 courage booster

Challenging situations at work sometimes cause stress levels to rocket. An important interview or giving a presentation can deplete your reserves, leaving you exhausted. This program will boost your energy and build confidence, so that you appear calm and perform well when it counts. Try to find somewhere quiet to practice.

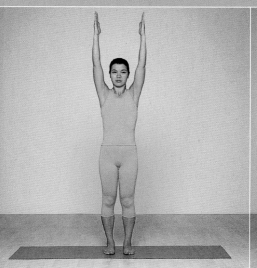

1 Standing Upward Stretch (see p.38)

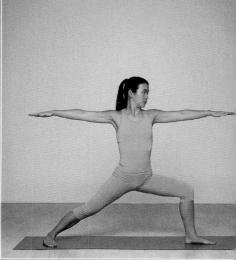

2 Side Warrior (see pp.52–53)

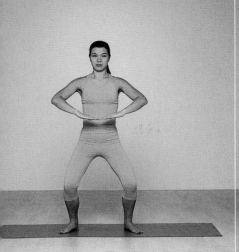

3 French Press Stretch (see p.35)

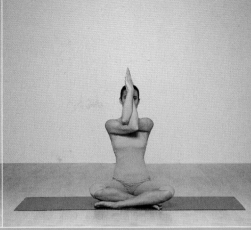

4 Eagle (see pp.44–45)

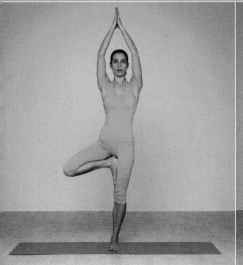

5 Tree (see pp.50–51)

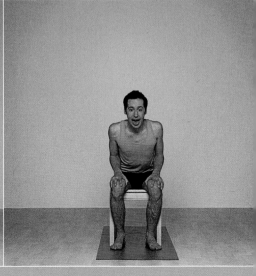

6 Roaring Lion (see pp.80–81)

tactics
4 survival

Sometimes it all gets too much – something triggers a sudden increase in your stress levels. This program is designed for such emergencies! These practices use your breath to enable you to become focused and centered, so you relax and regain your poise. Memorize the sequence, ready to recall when the need arises.

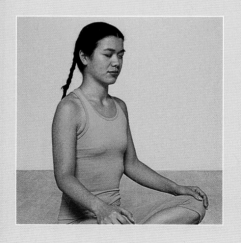

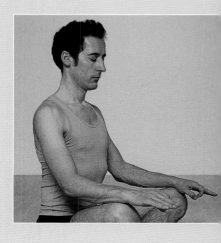

1 Instant Relaxation (see p.107)

2 Centering Mudra (see p.101)

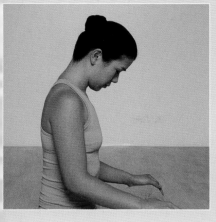

3 Neck Stretches (see pp.36–37)

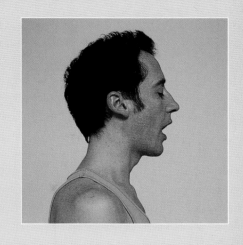

4 Audible Breath (see p.100)

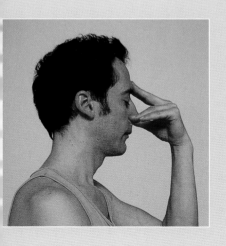

5 Alternate Nostril Breathing (see p.102)

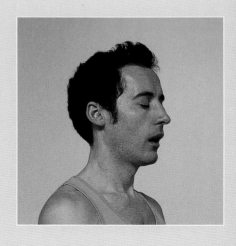

6 Sounds Breathing (see p.103)

⑤ after-work energizer

After work can sometimes be the only time you have to socialize with your friends; however, by the end of the day, it can be hard to find the energy to enjoy yourself. This program is designed to help you to let go of work problems, create some vitality, and still have enough time to freshen up before you leave the office!

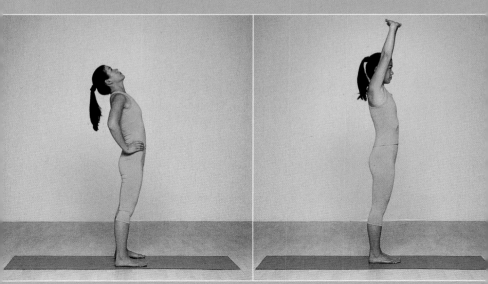

① Standing Back Arch (see p.40)

② Standing Arm Stretches (see p.34)

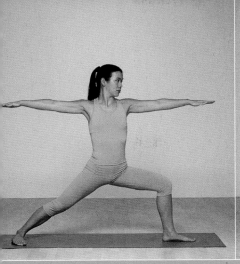

3 Side Warrior (see pp.52–53)

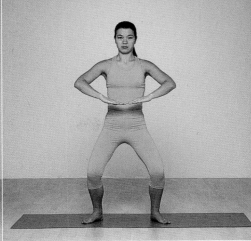

4 French Press Stretch (see p.35)

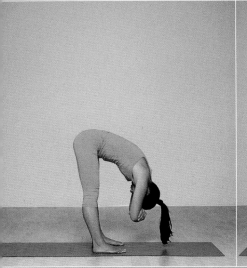

5 Forward Bend (see pp.48–49)

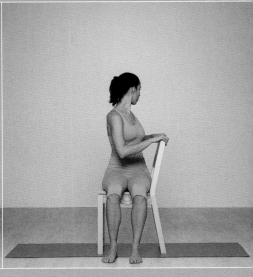

6 Chair Twist (see pp.98–99)

⑥ evening
pick-me-up

This program can be used to prepare you for the evening ahead when you have access to floor space and comfortable clothing. Back-arching postures release stress and raise your energy levels, helping you let go of the work of the day; the simple inversion restores your sense of inner calm while resting the legs.

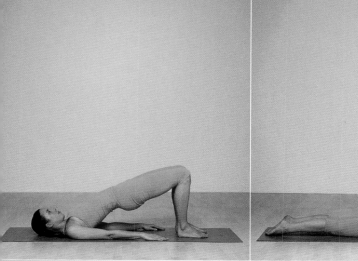

❶ Bridge (see pp.72–73)

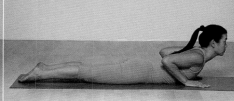

❷ Cobra (see pp.58–59)

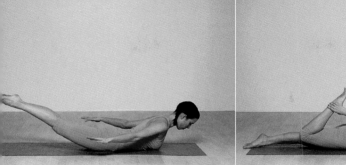

3 Locust (see pp.60–61)

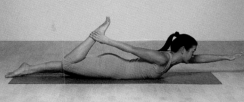

4 Half Bow (see pp.62–63)

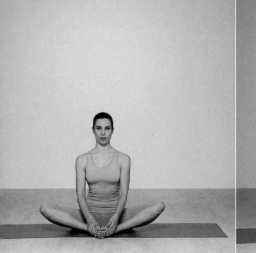

5 Cobbler (see pp.90–91)

6 Legs up the Wall (see pp.74–75)

7 evening
relaxer

If you are not going out for the evening, do this gentle, slow yoga practice at home, which will help you unwind and cast off all the accumulated stress of the day. These postures, practiced in harmony with the breath, are time-honored ways of relieving physical tension and releasing feelings of being under pressure.

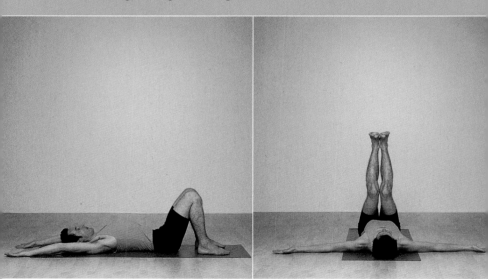

1 Supine Arms Over Head (see p.30)

2 Supine Legs Up Arms Out (see p.32)

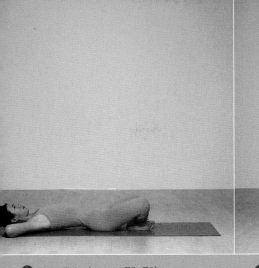

3 Easy Fish (see pp.78–79)

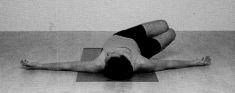

4 Supine Twist (see p.33)

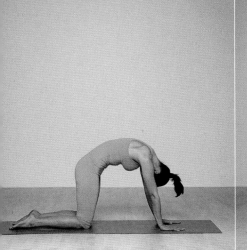

5 Cat (see pp.82–83)

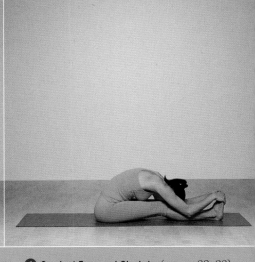

6 Seated Forward Stretch (see pp.88–89)

(8) weekend invigorator

Always try to build in some regular yoga time at the weekend. This program provides a longer practice, incorporating a balanced series of postures to open and stretch every part of your body. As you practice, you will feel your energy flowing more freely, while your general sense of wellbeing is enhanced and the mind calmed.

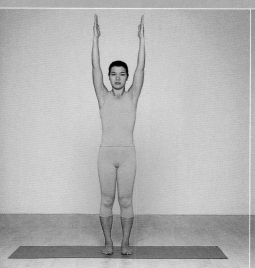

1 Standing Upward Stretch (see p.38)

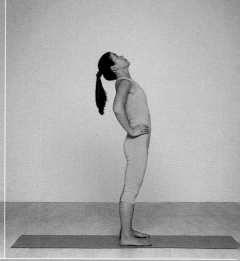

2 Standing Back Arch (see p.40)

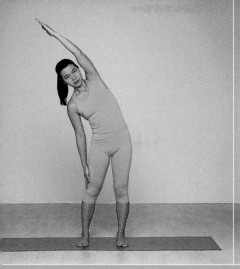

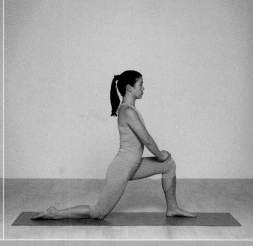

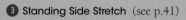
3 Standing Side Stretch (see p.41)

4 Lunge Warrior (see pp.54–55)

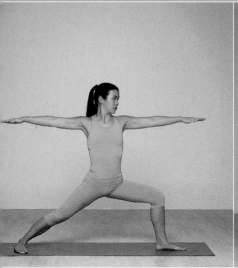

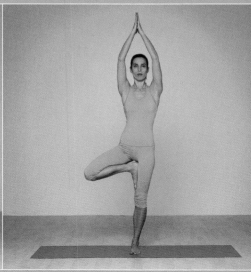

5 Side Warrior (see pp.52–53)

6 Tree (see pp.50–51) ▶

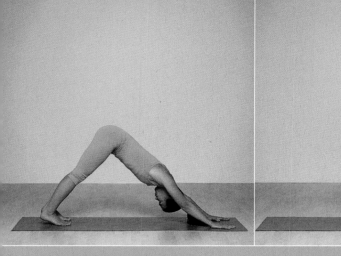

7 Downward Dog (see pp.56–57)

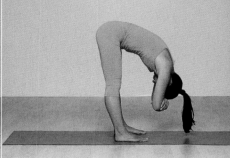

8 Forward Bend (see pp.48–49)

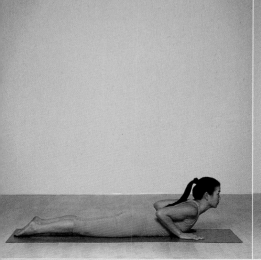

9 Cobra (see pp.58–59)

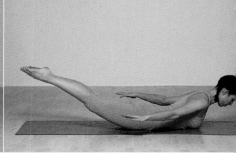

10 Locust (see pp.60–61)

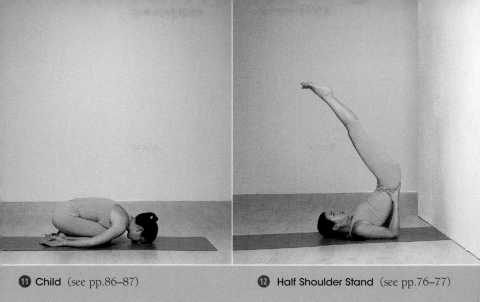

11 Child (see pp.86–87)

12 Half Shoulder Stand (see pp.76–77)

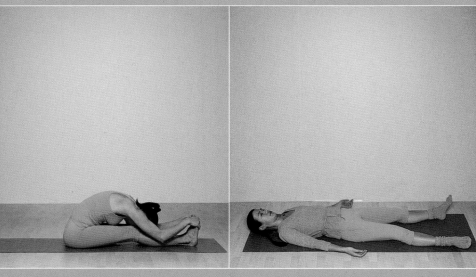

13 Seated Forward Stretch (see pp.88–89)

14 10-Minute Relaxation (see pp.108–109)

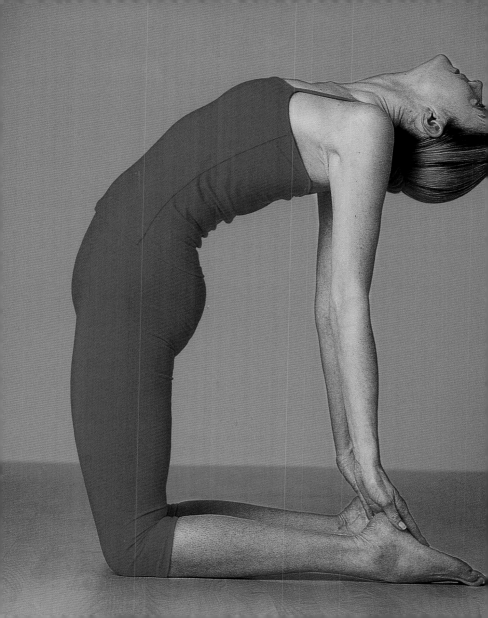

energetic

boosting
energy

The appeal of yoga is universal and timeless. Its holistic practices work on the physical, mental, emotional, and spiritual planes, boosting your energy levels and helping you live more positively.

Yoga is a tried-and-tested practical method of achieving all-around good health. It does not seek to offer a quick fix, but provides a long-term program for living positively. Its combination of physical postures, breathing practices, relaxation, meditation, and lifestyle guidance can help you stay physically fit and mentally alert, and live more positively and mindfully. For many people, yoga becomes a lifelong journey of self-discovery, bringing peace of mind and inner happiness.

Unlike some forms of exercise, yoga is suitable for everyone. Whatever your age or level of fitness, yoga is a very safe form of exercise provided you work within your limits. However, please read through the text in the box below, entitled "Health Concerns," before you begin, since some yoga practices can be physically demanding.

HEALTH CONCERNS

If a health practitioner has advised you not to overexert yourself physically, or if you have any other health concerns, seek advice from a qualified yoga therapist or teacher (see p.495) before using this book. Page 9 provides basic advice for some common medical conditions and, where appropriate, "Take Care" advice and "Alternatives" are given for individual practices. If you are pregnant, or have recently given birth, ask a suitably qualified yoga teacher which practices would be appropriate for you.

Life is energy

Human beings are complex energy systems, with energy processes taking place at physical, mental, emotional, and spiritual levels. The simplest form of energy is metabolic. This derives from the food we eat and the air we breathe. There is also vital energy – feeling glad to be alive and bursting with health.

For many people, vital energy is no more than an expression of the collective physical energies generated by the way mind and body work together. But for others it is the secret ingredient that makes the difference. In yoga, this vital energy is known as *prana*, the embodiment of the universal life force that flows everywhere and through everything – the "intelligence" behind creation.

Symptoms of low energy

Whatever you believe, everyone accepts that feeling good does not depend simply on how much energy you possess, but also on whether it is flowing freely. Sometimes energy becomes blocked, resulting in low levels of energy or an imbalance

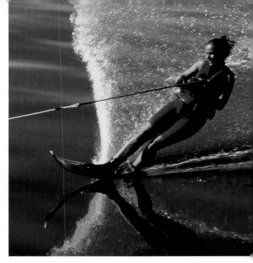

High energy levels give you a zest for life that makes you physically active, positive-thinking, and emotionally robust.

between physical, mental, and emotional energies.

If you are suffering from low levels of energy, you may find that, while you can cope with your normal day-to-day routine, anything that requires a little more effort tires you quickly. You may lack strength or stamina. Or you may have a general feeling of being physically "out of sorts" in which you wake up feeling tired.

Reduced energy levels may be expressed in poor postural habits and a lack of spring in your step. You may find that you are more susceptible to colds and other minor ailments. In extreme cases, you may find that virtually everything you do tires you or leaves you feeling weak.

Mentally, you may find that your concentration levels are so low that you find it difficult to keep your mind on your work, or to read a book or watch television without becoming distracted or bored. Remembering things and making decisions may be more difficult. You may find it difficult to raise much enthusiasm for doing anything at all.

At an emotional level, symptoms of low energy include becoming more easily irritated and upset, and more susceptible to anger, fear, jealousy, or envy. You may find yourself more critical of the world, your family, and your friends, and find it harder to accept change. As such negative emotions take hold, you become less able to laugh and to participate in and enjoy life. You become easily dragged down by events, tending to see problems rather than opportunities in new situations. Such feelings themselves drain you of energy.

Causes of low energy

The causes of low or out-of-balance energy levels are many and varied. There may be a single, identifiable cause, but more often there will be several factors contributing to your lack of energy, including:

- underlying medical conditions
- unbalanced diet
- sedentary lifestyle
- sleep deprivation
- stressful life situations.

Underlying medical conditions

Low energy levels may indicate an underlying medical problem. Conditions commonly associated with fatigue include depression, anxiety, and insomnia. Recovering from viral illnesses, anemia, low thyroid gland function, breathing problems such as severe asthma and hyperventilation, uncontrolled diabetes, and chronic pain (for example, back pain or arthritis) can also cause fatigue.

Prolonged fatigue may also be associated with more serious illnesses, so consult your doctor if you are worried.

Unbalanced diet

A well-balanced diet is essential
to high energy levels. Nutritional
inputs must keep pace with the
demands of metabolism, and both
undereating and overeating can
adversely affect energy levels. So
can eating over-processed food,
and foods that contain many artificial
additives and/or salt, sugar, or added
flavorings. Consuming excessive
quantities of foods that are potentially
addictive, such as those containing
caffeine and alcohol, also leads to
energy imbalances.

Sedentary lifestyle

Anyone who has been incapacitated
in some way for any length of time
will know how quickly muscle mass
and stamina can deteriorate through
lack of activity. However, it does not
necessarily take an accident or illness
to reduce your strength and stamina.

A sedentary lifestyle, often
accompanied by poor postural
habits, can adversely affect digestive
processes, reduce respiratory
capacity, place increased strain on
the cardiovascular system, and cause

YOGA AND EATING

Yoga encourages you to eat
moderately and simply, to eat
natural, fresh foods as far as possible,
and to pay attention to how you eat.
The guidelines below will help you
become more aware of your eating
habits. They will also help you digest
food more effectively.

- Eat freshly prepared meals.
- Do not eat until the last meal has
  been digested (up to three hours).
- Avoid distractions while eating,
  such as reading the newspaper or
  watching television.
- Do not eat when you are angry or
  upset about something.
- Take small mouthfuls and chew well.
- Do not drink large amounts of
  water (or other fluids) during meals.
- Drink plenty of water at other times.

muscle imbalances and weakness. In
addition, inactivity can cause mental
dullness, leading to a vicious circle of
mental and physical fatigue.

Sleep deprivation

Sleep deprivation is a common
problem (eight hours' sleep is about
the right amount for most people).
Unless a sleep debt is made up in the

following days, the debt grows. So, while you may superficially become used to an inadequate sleep regime, your immune system and the body's repair and "battery recharging" mechanisms suffer. This can result in poor reaction times, concentration, memory, and physical performance, and in poor judgment and frequent mood swings.

Our body rhythms can be upset by lifestyles that deviate strongly from the powerful sleep regulating stimuli of sunrise and nightfall. Shift workers are often affected, feeling drowsy at work and unable to sleep when they get home. At worst, digestive, cardiovascular, emotional, and mental problems may result.

Stressful life situations

Long hours spent at your workplace or heavy workloads, particularly if the work involves repetitive or boring tasks, can be draining both mentally and physically.

Bringing up a young family can be challenging, and combining it with a busy job inevitably adds to the pressures. Many people are continually working against the clock, trying to fit in as many tasks as possible. This can sap energy and result in a dependency on stimulants, such as nicotine, to help get through the day, and on alcohol to wind down at the end of it. The benefits of these substances are fleeting and the adverse effects long term.

In addition, financial worries, strained relationships, feeling lonely, and other personal problems can all reduce energy reserves, fostering a negative approach to life in general.

How yoga can help

The central purpose of yoga is to enable us to experience the limitless life energy that is the core of our being. Normally this is impossible because we are too enmeshed in the web of our daily lives. We tend to be too preoccupied with our desires, our attachment to objects and people, our prejudices and dislikes, and with the physical, mental, and emotional stresses that flow from them.

The way to overcome this limited way of living is to be able to "let go." Patanjali, a great yoga sage who lived over 2,000 years ago, described it as being able to "still the thought waves of the mind". Bringing the mind to a state of quiet calm is not easy, but it can be done by practicing the physical postures, breathing practices, relaxation, concentration, and meditation that together comprise the practice of yoga.

Practicing the physical postures brings improvements in cardiovascular endurance, muscle strength, flexibility, balance and coordination, and body reaction times. Gradually, your self-esteem and your life energy improve. Simply by regularly practicing the postures, you become generally more alive both physically and mentally.

Patanjali taught that we must change the habitual ways we think and act. He offered guidance on how we should relate to other people and to the world around us with a set of

MAXIMS FOR LIVING

A positive relationship with the world and with yourself was of fundamental importance to Patanjali. Try to live by his maxims (interpreted below). They will help you live more positively, allowing life energy to flow more freely through you.

In your relationship with the world around you, you should:

• Avoid causing harm; endeavor to be compassionate.

• Be honest in all your thoughts, words, and actions.

• Never steal from others. This applies not only to possessions, but also to wasting other people's time, energy, and goodwill.

• Be faithful and selfless in all your personal relationships.

• Avoid acquiring or holding on to material things (or people) for the sake of it, or for selfish reasons.

In relation to yourself, you should work to:

• Develop purity in mind, body, and spirit – inner and outer cleanliness.

• Pursue simplicity in life, and try to make the most of whatever life brings.

• Develop physical and mental resolve (through yoga practices) to withstand difficulties and disappointments in life.

• Learn to identify with your inner self rather than with your habitual ways of acting and seeing situations.

• Accept that there is more to life than the material world, and be respectful of the intelligence underpinning life.

personal observances designed to encourage a healthy, positive approach to life. In essence, he taught mindfulness: "being with what is." This means giving all of your attention to whomever you are with or whatever you are doing, and not allowing yourself to be carried away by some distracting train of thought or letting your emotions cloud your sense of judgment.

New approach to life

Because most of us are used to living in ways that put our egos, our desires and attachments, our prejudices, and our hopes and fears at the center, letting go and acting in a selfless manner is difficult. And it is not just a question of the actions themselves, but the spirit in which they are done; we need to enjoy our selfless actions, not do them grudgingly.

If you are able to let go of negative attitudes and emotions, rather than giving way to them or suppressing them; if you respect others, show compassion, and learn to follow your heart, then you will find that your energy levels naturally rise. And you will become less susceptible to being worn down by the negativity of others. These are not changes that can be achieved overnight. You must work at them consistently, trying to be more objective and more discriminating, and to consciously cultivate positive attitudes.

Take one of Patanjali's principles of behavior and attitude (see "Maxims for Living," p.137), and

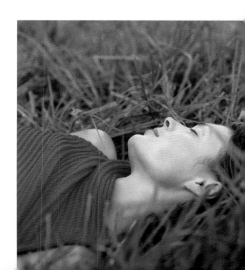

Go for a walk in the country or by the sea and reflect on your attitudes and behavior toward others. Meditate on the beauty and the stillness of nature.

observe how close you get to it in your thoughts, intentions, and actions during the course of a day. The next day, make a positive effort to behave in accordance with the same principle, and observe the difference in the way you feel when you do. Work your way through all the maxims in this fashion. Provided you work with determination and are not discouraged by setbacks, you will find yourself gradually becoming more aware, more mindful, more energized – and happier!

Trying to be more in tune with nature and finding more time for yourself can help, too. Paying attention to, and appreciating, the world around you, and marvelling at the wonders of nature, can be especially helpful in enabling you to appreciate the intelligence underlying the universe, and to be less self-centered. Last, if you can spend time in the countryside or open spaces, away from the activity, noise, and pollution of modern society, you can benefit energetically simply from the quietness and the improved quality of the air you breathe.

HOW TO USE THIS SECTION

Energetic is divided into three sub-sections. **Foundations** provides guidance on doing yoga and some basic breathing and preliminary stretches. Familiarize yourself with these first before moving on to **Building Blocks**. This contains a selection of postures and breathing practices, as well as a simple meditation and relaxation technique. Work through these postures gradually, selecting one or two to work on at a time, rather than trying to do them all at once. Look at the photographs first to get a feel for the overall shape of the posture. Then follow the accompanying step-by-step instructions carefully. If you find a posture difficult to do, try the alternative, if one is given.

Programs combines selected postures and other practices in a series of short yoga programs designed for particular situations and needs. Make sure that you understand how to do the postures first before trying these programs.

Yoga is traditionally learned from a teacher, and you will benefit from going to a class, if you are not already doing so. Organizations that can help you find a qualified teacher are listed on page 495.

the basics

In yoga, basic standing, sitting, and lying down positions are important in their own right, helping you to develop stability and awareness of the benefits of alignment for your posture, your breathing, and for the free flow of energy. They also provide the foundations from which other postures are developed.

In addition, being able to sit comfortably and steadily is important for breathing practices and also for meditation, helping you remain focused without distractions from physical tensions. Lying down is often used to develop body and breath awareness, and to relax and let your body absorb the beneficial effects of other yoga practices.

If you find it impossible to achieve the full posture, it can be very helpful to use a prop, such as a block or cushion, ensure that you do not strain your body.

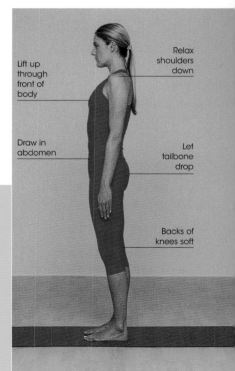

Lift up through front of body

Draw in abdomen

Relax shoulders down

Let tailbone drop

Backs of knees soft

STANDING

Stand up straight with your feet parallel, hip-width apart, and your ears, tops of shoulders, hips, and ankles in line. Press your feet to the ground and lift upwards through your body. Broaden across the top of the chest. Feel yourself balanced in every direction, head as if suspended by a thread from the ceiling. Look straight ahead, relax, and breathe easily.

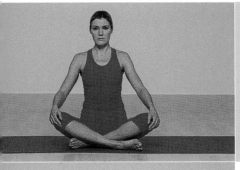

EASY SITTING

This basic posture is good for breathing practices. Cross your shins with each foot under the opposite calf or knee. Position yourself on the front edge of your sitting bones, with the spine long and the head erect. Relax the shoulders. If your knees are higher than your hips, sit on a block or another support.

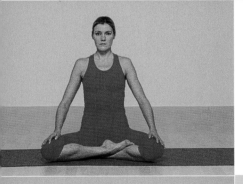

ADVANCED SITTING

If you are fairly flexible, this is a more stable position for prolonged sitting (for example, in meditation). Sit with your legs spread. Bring the sole of your left foot against the inside of your right thigh and your right foot on to, or in front of, your left calf, with the heels touching. Your knees should be resting on the floor. Do not strain to sit in the posture.

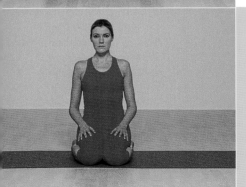

KNEELING

Try this position if you find basic cross-legged sitting uncomfortable. Sit on your heels with the tops of your thighs facing the ceiling. Alternatively, if you are going to stay longer, position your knees and feet hip-width apart and sit on blocks, a folded blanket, or a bolster. Keep your spine long and your head erect, with the shoulders and the neck relaxed.

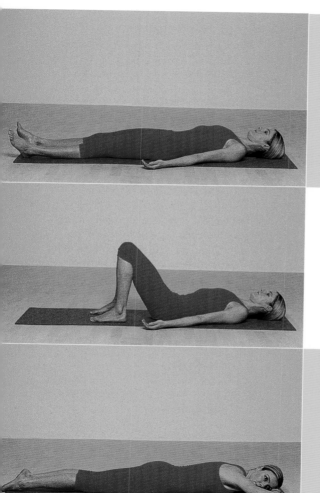

LYING ON BACK

Lie with your legs stretched out, feet hip-width apart. Allow the feet and legs to roll out. Place your arms away from the body, backs of the hands on the floor. Relax the neck and rest the center of the back of the head on the floor.

LYING WITH LEGS BENT

If you feel any discomfort in your lower back when lying flat, having your legs bent can be a good alternative. Keep your feet hip-width apart and let the knees rest against each other.

LYING ON FRONT

Between prone postures you might like to relax by lying on your front. Keep your feet hip-width apart and use the backs of your hands as a pillow on which to rest your turned head. Let the legs relax and the heels fall outwards.

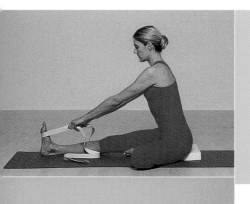

USING BELTS AND BLOCKS

Belts and blocks can be used in a wide variety of situations as supports and stabilizers to help you practice postures effectively without straining yourself. For example, in forward-bending movements – as shown here – using a belt helps protect the back if you have tight hamstrings or tight hips.

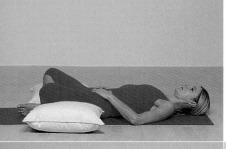

USING PILLOWS

Pillows can be used to support different parts of the body. Here they are shown supporting the thighs in Supine Butterfly (see p.216), allowing the inner and the outer thigh muscles to relax, the hips to open farther, and the person to stay in the posture longer without being distracted by discomfort.

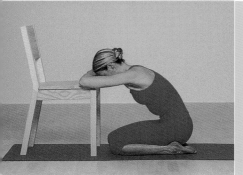

USING A CHAIR

Chairs can be used to modify postures. Shown here is a version of Child (see p.198) for someone with HBP. A chair can also be used for breathing or meditation practices if sitting or kneeling on the floor is uncomfortable. Sit toward the front of the chair, with the soles of the feet flat on the floor (or block), hands resting on the thighs or in the lap.

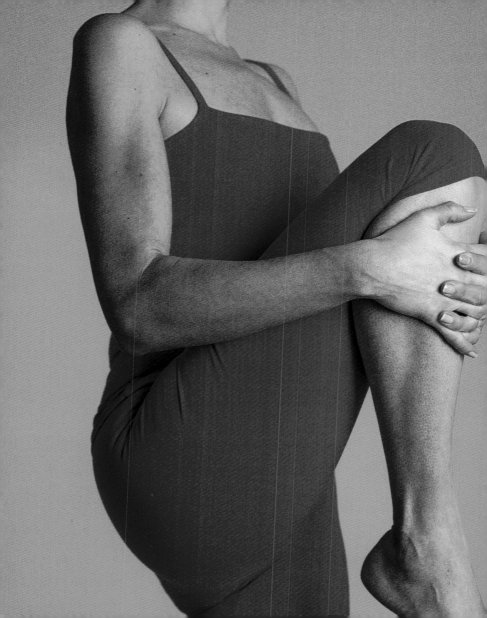

foundations

This section provides advice for those new to yoga. It includes basic standing, sitting, and lying positions; preliminary practices to bring awareness to your yoga practice, and breathe-and-stretch exercises to loosen the body and help coordinate breath with movement.

centering

Take a few minutes before starting your yoga practice to settle the mind and body by focusing on the here and now. This technique is known as centering, and helps develop awareness and mindfulness.

You can center yourself by standing, sitting, or lying down quietly for a few minutes in a comfortable position. Simply observe your breath, letting it settle into a quiet, natural rhythm. As you do so, the activity in your mind will lessen. However, if your body is stiff and your muscles tense, you will find the following lying down centering relaxation practice helpful before starting to do the postures.

lying down centering

1 Lie on the floor with your knees bent, feet hip-width apart. Place your arms away from the sides of the body, the backs of the hands on the floor, and the fingers gently curling inward. Position the center of the back of the head on the floor, and relax the neck. If your neck feels strained, try placing a small support (for example, a block, thin pillow, or folded blanket) underneath your head.

2 Allow your lower back to sink toward the floor. Slide your feet along the floor to stretch the legs out. Let the legs relax and the feet fall outward. (If you feel discomfort in your back, keep your knees bent.) Close your eyes. Be aware of how balanced your body feels. Are the different parts of the body sinking into the floor equally, or are there tensions or restrictions in some areas?

3 Slowly take your attention to each part of your body, starting with the feet and working upward through the lower legs, upper legs, hips, buttocks, hands, lower arms, upper arms, chest, lower back, shoulders, neck, and face. Ask each part of the body to relax and allow them all to release down into the floor. Become aware of your breath and make sure you are breathing through your nostrils. Do not try to control the breath or change it in any way; simply observe its movement in and out of the body. Let your breath settle into a slow, deep, natural rhythm. Each time you breathe out be aware of letting go. Feel the body "sinking" into the floor, while at the same time it is supported by the floor.

4 Bring your attention to your out-breath. Allow it to become a little longer than your in-breath. Now count down 10 out-breaths. The breath should remain calm and unhurried as you count. When you reach zero, gently turn the head from side to side three times. Then, on an in-breath, stretch your arms up to the ceiling and then behind you. Stretch through to the fingertips as you press your lower back to the floor and your heels gently toward the wall in front of you. Relax into the stretch for a few breaths. Then, on an out-breath, bring your arms back down to your sides, or to rest on your abdomen, and let go completely. Gently turn onto one side of your body, pause for a moment, then slowly sit or stand up.

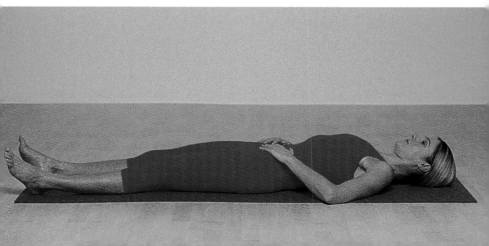

basic
breathing

There is a fundamental connection between the breath and your physical, mental, and emotional states. The breath is the pathway for *prana* – "the breath behind the breath" – to enter the body.

Breathing provides oxygen for the metabolic processes from which we derive the energy to move, think, and feel, and carries away carbon dioxide, the main waste product of metabolism. Physical tension in the respiratory muscles between and around the ribs can cause tightness in the chest, and even chest pain. Relaxed breathing techniques will release tension from the whole of the upper body, including the neck and shoulders. This will improve your ability to adjust your breathing to meet changing requirements.

The breath also provides a powerful link between mind and body. By controlling your breathing patterns – for example, the rhythm and depth of breathing, the length of the out-breath, and the balance between right and left nostrils – you can influence your physical, mental, and emotional states.

Good breathing habits

Yoga encourages breathing through the nose, full use of the diaphragm, a slow, smooth breathing pattern, and coordination of movement and breath. In the poses, opening movements, such as backbends, are usually done on an in-breath and closing movements, such as forward bends, on an out-breath.

The breathing practice opposite will help develop awareness of the respiratory muscles and encourage good breathing habits. It can also be done standing or lying down.

sitting sectional breathing

Sectional breathing helps unlock energy blocks associated with poor breathing habits. After completing

Step 3, combine all three steps to produce full, continuous in-breaths and out-breaths.

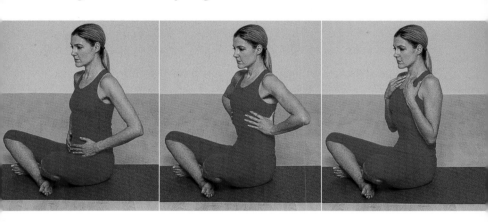

1 Sit comfortably with your palms resting on your abdomen, the middle fingers just touching. Breathe into your hands, feeling the abdomen swell out and the fingers move apart as you breathe in. Then feel the abdomen sink back as you exhale. Take six even breaths.

2 Bring your hands to your ribcage, with your fingers to the front and thumbs on the back ribs. Feel the ribs expand into the hands on the in-breath and then relax back inward as you exhale. Take six breaths, keeping the abdomen as still as possible.

3 Rest the fronts of your fingers just below your collar bones. Breathe in, feeling the top of the chest expand and the fingers and shoulders rise up toward the head. As you breathe out, feel the fingers sink back down. Take six breaths.

breathe and
stretch

The following exercises work on coordinating movement with the breath, and stretching tight muscles. Being aware of your breath as you move will allow energy to flow more freely through your body.

up and down stretch

1 Assume the basic standing position (see p.140) with your feet parallel and about hip-width apart. Looking straight ahead, take several full breaths.

2 On an in-breath, sweep your arms slowly out to the side and up above your head. Bring your palms together, fingers pointing toward the ceiling. Continue to look straight ahead.

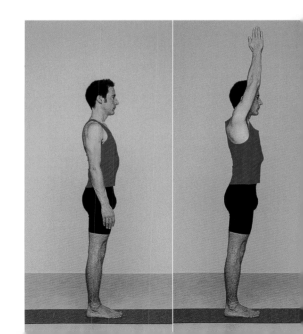

3 As you breathe out, fold the arms backward, bringing your palms together and hands down your back so that your fingers point toward the floor. At the same time, stretch your elbows toward the ceiling.

4 Interlock your fingers. As you breathe in, straighten out the arms again, stretching the palms of the hands up toward the ceiling.

5 Breathe out, sweeping your arms out to the sides and down. Breathe in as you take your arms back toward the wall behind you, interlocking the fingers again behind your back. Open your chest and hold in your abdomen.

6 Breathe out as you fold forward from the hips, with knees bent. Stretch the backs of the hands toward the ceiling. Come back up as you breathe in, stretching the arms back again. Lower the arms to the sides on the out-breath. Repeat the sequence several times.

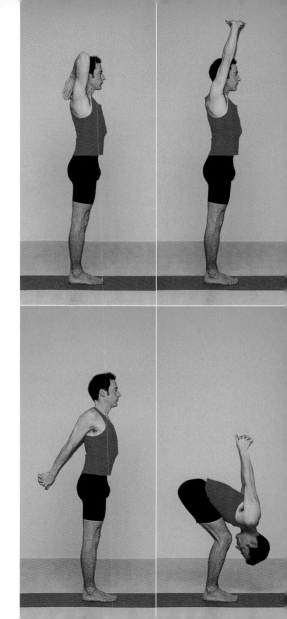

swimming breaststroke

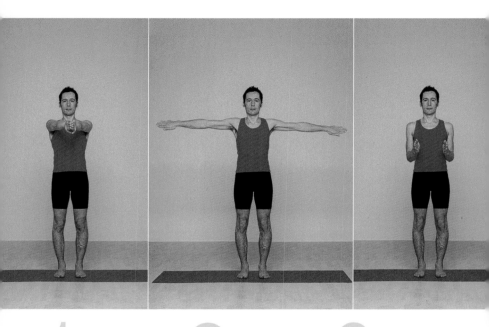

1 Stand up straight, feet parallel and hip-width apart. Stretch your arms forward at shoulder level, palms together. Take two or three breaths, then, on an in-breath, turn your palms out to bring the backs of the hands together.

2 As you breathe out, sweep the arms out to the side, then back and down to your sides in a circular motion, mimicking the arm movement of the breaststroke.

3 Keeping the elbows close to the sides of the body, stretch the arms forward and bring the palms together on the in-breath. Repeat the sequence several times, keeping the movement smooth and flowing.

swimming backstroke

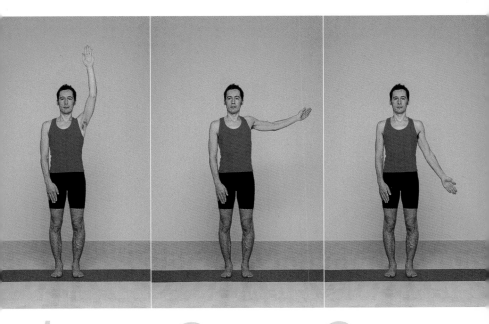

1 Stand up tall, feet parallel and hip-width apart. Place the palms of your hands on the fronts of your thighs. Let the breath settle into a regular rhythm. As you breathe in, bring your left arm forward and up toward the ceiling.

2 Continue in a circular motion, bringing your left arm behind you, as though swimming the backstroke. Press the right palm against the thigh to stop the body from twisting. Keep looking straight ahead of you.

3 Bring the arm down and forward. On the out-breath, circle the right arm back and down in the same way. Repeat several times. Then breathe in as you circle the right arm back and breathe out as you circle the left arm.

side bend and twist

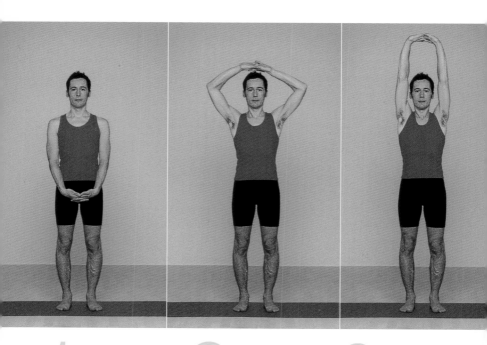

1 Assume the basic standing position, feet hip-width apart. Bring the hands together in front of the body and interlock the fingers. Take several breaths.

2 On an in-breath, roll the hands up the front of the body to bring them just above the head, with the palms facing the ceiling.

3 As you breathe out, stretch your palms toward the ceiling, keeping the shoulders down away from the ears. Lengthen through the arms.

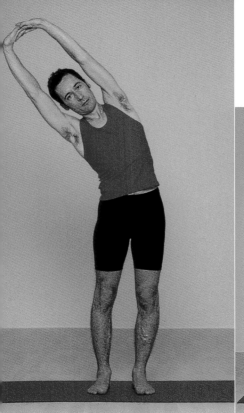

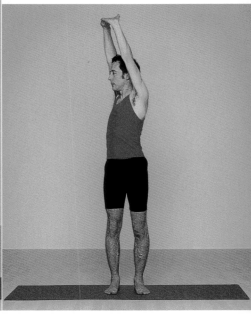

Breathe in, then, as you breathe out, bend to the right, hinging at the waist. Breathe in as you come back up to the center. As you breathe out, bend to the left, and breathe in as you come back up again.

Breathe out as you twist to the right, keeping the palms pushing towards the ceiling. Breathe in as you come back to face the front. Breathing out, twist to the left and come back to face the front again on the in-breath. Lower your arms in front of you as you breathe out, keeping the fingers interlocked. Repeat the entire sequence twice.

one-legged stretch

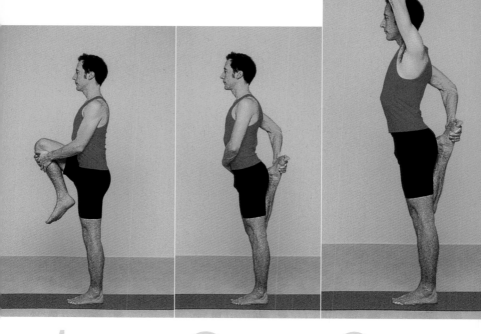

1 From the basic standing position, raise your right knee toward your chest and clasp your hands around the shin. Ease the knee toward the chest and take three slow, deep breaths.

2 Slide the right hand down to the foot and lower the knee. Press the heel against the right buttock. Place your left hand on the right hip. Take three breaths as you press the right hip forward against your left hand.

3 Stretch the left arm up beside the head. Take three breaths. Keeping the bent knee in line with the straight leg, release the right foot and slowly lower it to the floor. Repeat with the left leg.

knee lifts and kicks

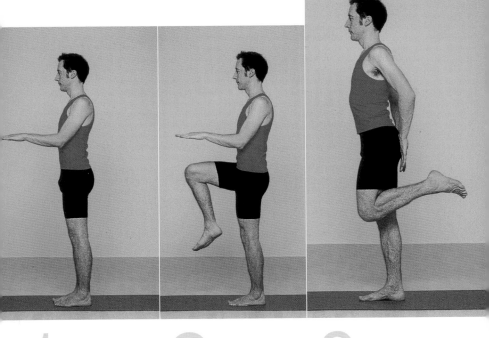

1 Assume the basic standing position, feet hip-width apart. Hold both hands out in front of you at waist level, palms facing the floor, elbows against the sides of your body. Let your breath settle into a smooth rhythm.

2 Alternately lift the right and left knee to touch the palms of the hands. Do not lower the arm or bend forward to meet the knee as it comes up. Start slowly, and gradually increase your speed.

3 Rest the backs of your hands on the buttocks. Alternately kick each leg back to touch the palm of the hand with the heel. Start slowly, gradually increasing speed. Repeat Steps 2 and 3 until slightly out of breath.

wide-legged squat

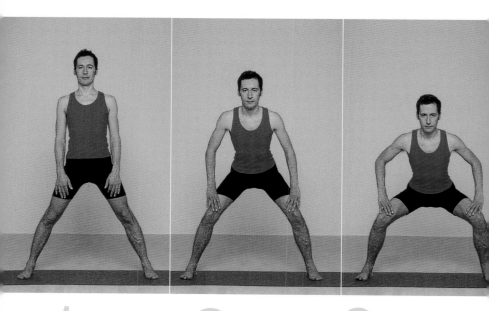

1 Stand upright with your legs about 3–4 ft (90–120 cm) apart, feet turned out a little, and knees in line with the toes. Look straight ahead.

2 Bend the knees slightly and bring your hands onto the insides of your thighs, just above your knees. Spread the fingers slightly and place the thumbs on the outside of the thighs. Take a breath in.

3 As you exhale, take your hips back as though you were going to sit down. Keep your spine long and do not let your hips sink below your knees. Come back up on the in-breath. Repeat slowly up to 10 times.

wide-legged lunge

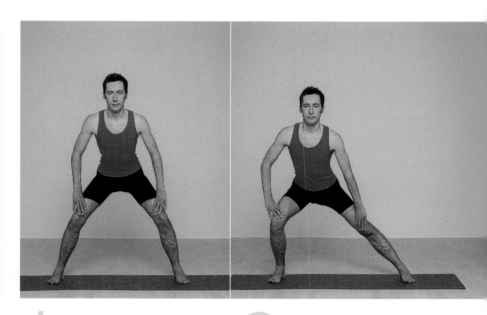

Stand with your knees slightly bent and your hands resting on the insides of your thighs just above the knees. Spread the fingers slightly and place the thumbs on the outside of the thighs. Take several breaths.

As you breathe out, lunge to the right, bending the right knee and straightening the left leg. Then lunge to the left as you breathe in. Repeat slowly up to 10 times, breathing out as you go to the left and in as you go to the right. Feel the stretch on the insides of the thighs. Make sure the bent knee stays in line with the toes.

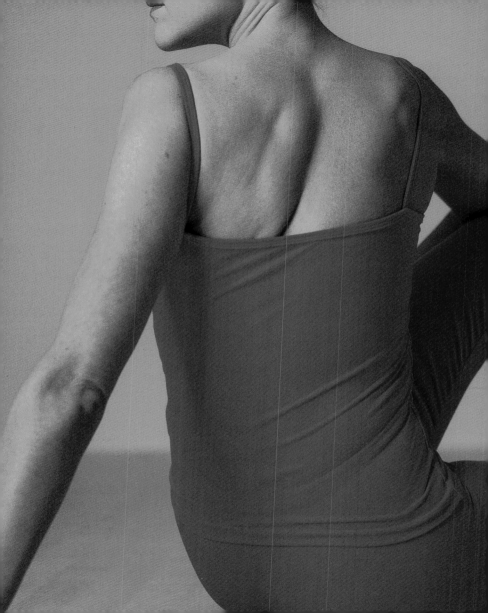

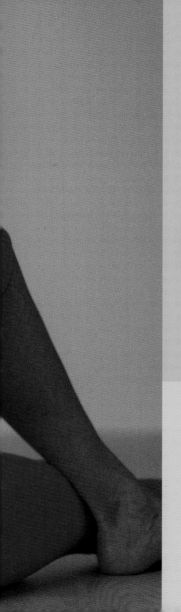

building blocks

This section presents a selection of postures and other yoga practices to revitalize your body, mind, and spirit. Stay in the postures only for as long as you are able to hold them steadily and comfortably, breathing evenly. Listen to your body as you practice and you will soon feel the benefits.

forward bend

Take the weight off your shoulders and allow the spine to stretch with this calming posture. Keep the feet rooted and the sitting bones lifting up to help stretch tight hamstrings. Come out slowly and carefully.

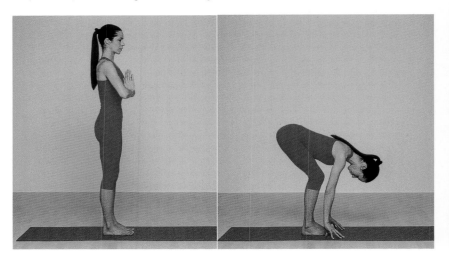

1 Assume the basic standing position (see p.140). Then bring the palms together in front of your chest in prayer position. Take several breaths, feeling yourself growing taller and becoming more relaxed.

2 As you breathe out, fold forward from the hips, bending your knees at the same time. Place your fingertips on the floor. Let the upper body rest on the thighs and keep the back long. Breathe easily.

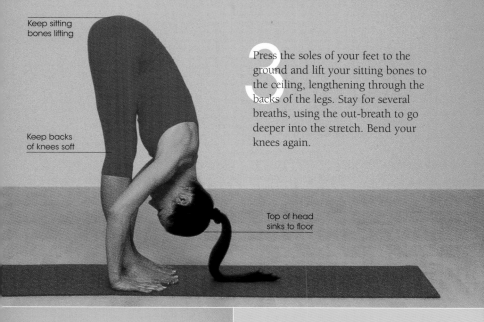

Keep sitting bones lifting

Keep backs of knees soft

Top of head sinks to floor

3 Press the soles of your feet to the ground and lift your sitting bones to the ceiling, lengthening through the backs of the legs. Stay for several breaths, using the out-breath to go deeper into the stretch. Bend your knees again.

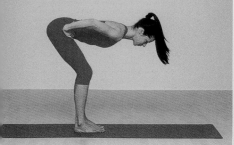

4 Put your hands on your hips and come up halfway on an in-breath. Lengthen through the spine on the out-breath. On an in-breath, hinging from the hips and keeping your back straight, come all the way up.

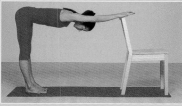

ALTERNATIVE

If you have HBP, a heart condition, glaucoma, or a detached retina, do a Half Forward Bend, resting your hands on the back or seat of a chair. Keep the abdomen gently pulled back towards the spine and the chest lifted. If you have lower back pain or sciatica, keep your knees bent.

warrior

This strong standing pose builds strength in the legs and back. Keep the tailbone dropping as you lift out of the hips toward the hands. Breathe evenly, remaining balanced and focused throughout.

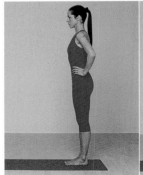 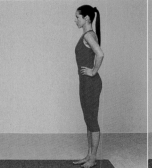 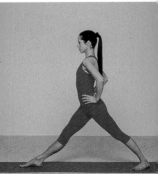

1 Stand with your feet together. Place your hands on your hips. Focus on your breath.

2 Pivoting on your heel, turn your left foot out about 45 degrees. Lift upward out of your hips as you breathe in.

3 As you exhale, take a large step forward with the right foot. Square the hips to the front, adjusting the position of your back foot if necessary. Take a breath in.

TAKE CARE

• If you have back problems, be cautious as you move into the final position. • Don't look up if you have neck problems. • If you have HBP or a heart condition, hold for a short time and keep your hands on your hips.

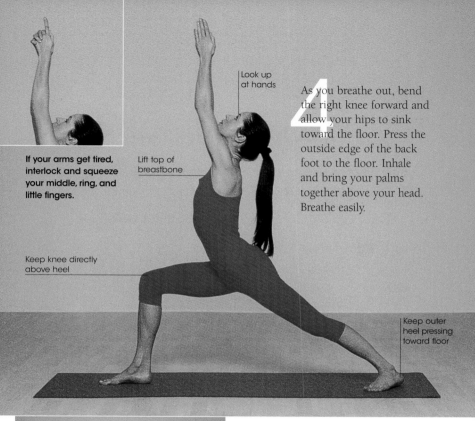

If your arms get tired, interlock and squeeze your middle, ring, and little fingers.

Look up at hands

Lift top of breastbone

Keep knee directly above heel

Keep outer heel pressing toward floor

4 As you breathe out, bend the right knee forward and allow your hips to sink toward the floor. Press the outside edge of the back foot to the floor. Inhale and bring your palms together above your head. Breathe easily.

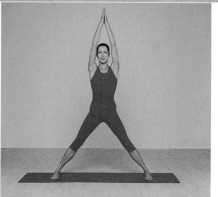

5 On an in-breath, straighten the right leg. Turn 90 degrees to come into a wide-legged position. Step your feet together and lower your arms. Repeat the sequence, turning the right foot out at Step 2 and stepping forward with the left foot at Step 3.

lunge
warrior

Lunge Warrior provides a powerful stretch through the thigh and hip of the back leg, extends the spine, and opens the chest. Feel the energy building as you breathe deeply into the ribcage.

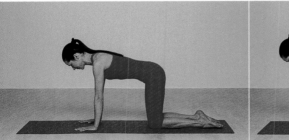
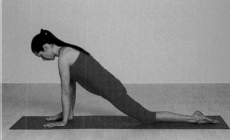

1 Begin on all fours with the hands directly beneath the shoulders and the knees beneath the hips. With fingers spread, press the palms to the floor, stretch through the arms, and bring the shoulders away from the ears.

2 As you exhale, take your right leg forward between your hands, so your knee is directly above the heel of your right foot. If necessary, come up onto your fingertips.

TAKE CARE
- If you have back problems, stop at Step 3 or 4 to begin with.
- Do not take the neck back at Step 6 if you have neck problems.
- If you have heart problems or HBP, stop at Step 4 or 5 and hold the position briefly.

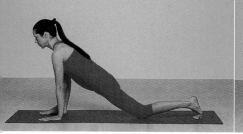

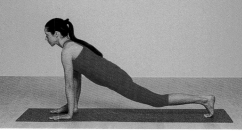

3 Tuck the toes of the left foot under and step the foot back a little. Let the right buttock sink toward the floor. Raise your head to look at the floor in front of you.

4 As you breathe in, extend the left heel backward and, for a stronger stretch, bring the knee off the floor. Lengthen through the upper body and look straight ahead.

5 Letting the knee hover just above the ground, place your hands on your right thigh and, as you breathe in, peel your upper body up, hinging at the hip. Breathe steadily. ▶

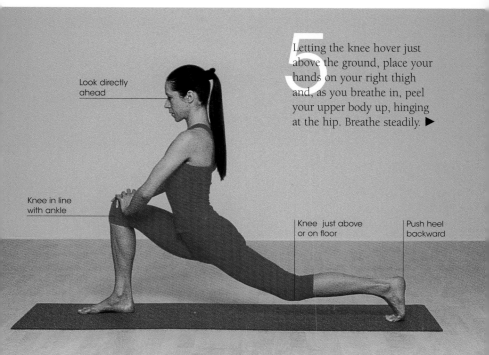

Look directly ahead

Knee in line with ankle

Knee just above or on floor

Push heel backward

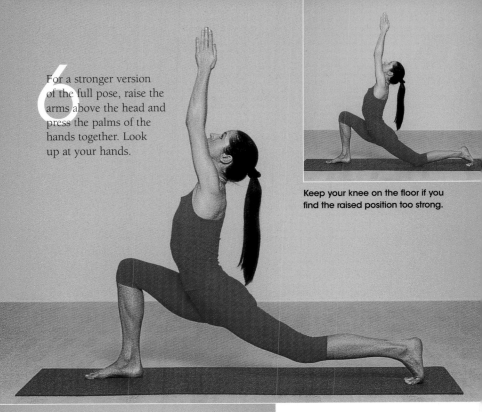

6 For a stronger version of the full pose, raise the arms above the head and press the palms of the hands together. Look up at your hands.

Keep your knee on the floor if you find the raised position too strong.

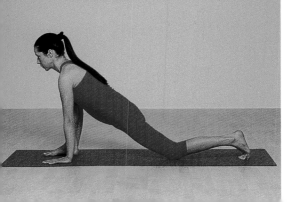

7 On an out-breath, fold forward and lower your hands to the floor on each side of your right foot. Bring your left knee to the floor. Gaze at the floor slightly ahead.

Come onto the front of your left foot. Look down at the floor and move your hips back to stretch through the back of the right leg. You may need to let your hands slide back as you move the hips back.

On an out-breath, take your right foot back to come into an all-fours position again. Your wrists should be positioned directly below your shoulders and your knees aligned with your hips. Look down at the floor.

Keeping your hands still, sit back on your heels on an out-breath, feeling the stretch through the spine. Relax the arms and stay for several breaths. Repeat Steps 1 to 9 on the left side of the body.

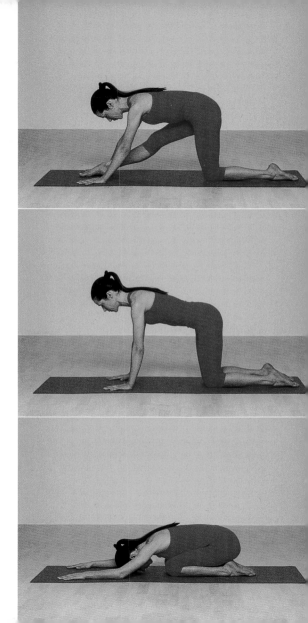

downward
dog

This calming inversion balances the upper and lower body. Keep
your weight moving up and back, your shoulders broad and soft,
as you stretch from the base of your fingers to your sitting bones.

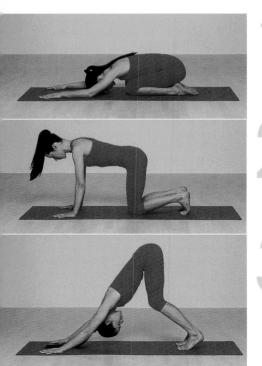

1 Sit on your heels with your legs hip-width apart. Fold your body forward on an out-breath. Stretch your arms forward and spread the fingers.

2 Breathing in, come up onto all fours, with the knees beneath the hips, the feet hip-width apart, and the hands shoulder-width apart. Press the palms into the floor and stretch through the arms. Tuck your toes under.

3 On an out-breath, lift your hips up and back. Keeping your knees bent, take your weight back toward your feet to lengthen through the spine. If your shoulders are tight, take your hands farther forward or your feet back to lengthen through the spine.

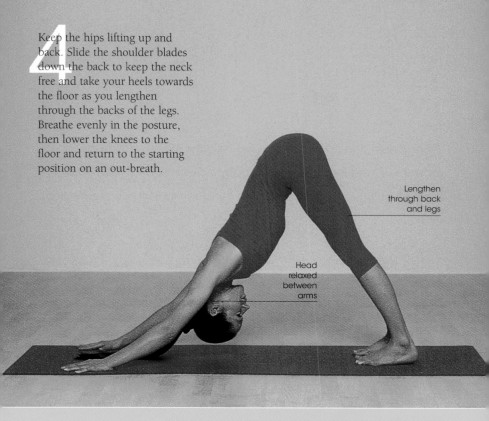

4 Keep the hips lifting up and back. Slide the shoulder blades down the back to keep the neck free and take your heels towards the floor as you lengthen through the backs of the legs. Breathe evenly in the posture, then lower the knees to the floor and return to the starting position on an out-breath.

Lengthen through back and legs

Head relaxed between arms

ALTERNATIVES

If you have HBP, a heart condition, glaucoma, or a detached retina, do the posture with your hands resting on a chair seat or back. If you have a back problem, do the posture cautiously with your knees bent throughout.

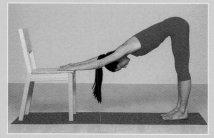

crocodile

This challenging static posture uses muscles in the arms, back, abdomen, and legs to keep the body balanced and still. In the posture, stay focused and visualize the body floating above the floor.

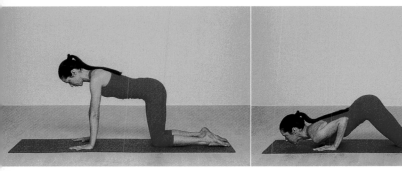

1 Start on all fours with your knees beneath your hips, your hands a little in front of your shoulders, and your feet hip-width apart. Look down. Take several breaths.

2 On an out-breath, bend your arms and lower your upper body towards the floor. Stop when your chest is a few inches above the floor. Keep your elbows tucked in close to the side of your body.

TAKE CARE
If you are very overweight, or have HBP or a heart condition, hold the full pose for a short time only or try the alternative posture (right).

3 Breathing in, tuck your toes under and lift your knees off the floor. Take the top of your chest forward, so that your elbows are above your wrists. Pull your abdomen back toward the spine, so your whole body is parallel to the floor. Step your feet back if you need to.

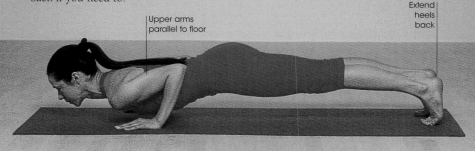

Upper arms parallel to floor

Extend heels back

4 To come out of the pose, lower the knees back to the floor on an out-breath. Then slowly lower the rest of the body to the floor. Rest with your head on the backs of your hands. Come back into the all-fours position and repeat the sequence once.

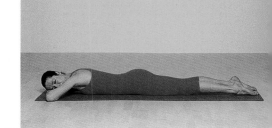

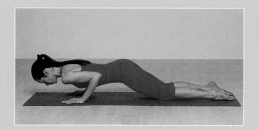

ALTERNATIVE

If you cannot hold your body parallel to the floor in the final position, practice with your knees on the floor until you are stronger.

upward dog

This posture gives a powerful upward lift through the front of the body, extending the spine and opening the chest to encourage ribcage breathing. It gives you a feeling of strength and vitality.

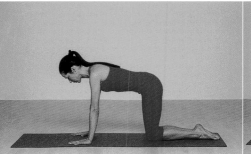
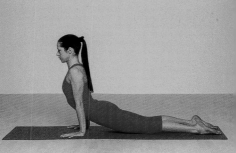

1 Start on your hands and knees, arms shoulder-width apart, feet and knees a little apart. Spread your fingers, with the middle finger pointing directly ahead. Take several breaths.

2 Breathe in deeply and, as you breathe out, allow your hips to sink forward and down. Keep your arms straight, insides of elbows facing each other, and look straight ahead. Roll the shoulders back and down.

TAKE CARE
- If you have HBP or a heart condition, hold the posture for short time only.
- Stretch forward cautiously if you have a hernia, or have had recent abdominal surgery, or suffer back pain.

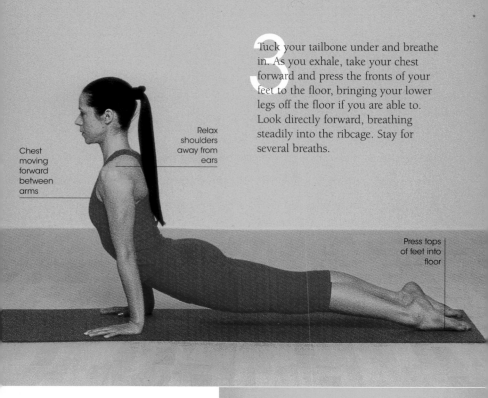

3 Tuck your tailbone under and breathe in. As you exhale, take your chest forward and press the fronts of your feet to the floor, bringing your lower legs off the floor if you are able to. Look directly forward, breathing steadily into the ribcage. Stay for several breaths.

Chest moving forward between arms

Relax shoulders away from ears

Press tops of feet into floor

4 To come out of the pose, bend the arms to lower yourself to the floor. Lie on your front, arms beside your body, palms facing up, resting with your head turned to the side.

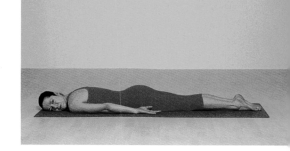

sun salute

This dynamic sequence energizes the whole body system. Focus on coordinating movement with breath and making the sequence fluid. Repeat three times at first, building up in multiples of three.

1 Stand up straight with your feet together, and your palms together in prayer position in front of your chest. Look straight ahead. Center yourself and then inhale fully.

2 As you exhale, open the palms and lower your hands to bring the arms to the sides of the body. Gently stretch the fingers toward the floor.

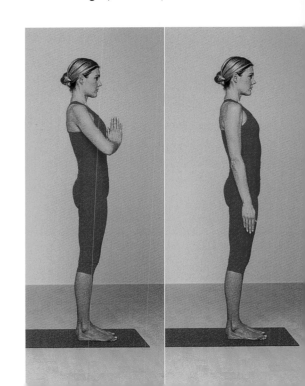

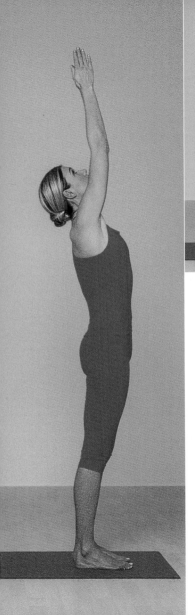
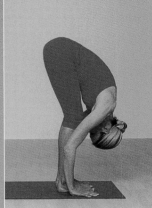
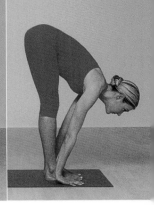

3 As you inhale, turn the palms out and circle your arms out to the side and up above your head. Bring your palms together and stretch up as you slightly arch backward. Look up at your hands.

4 Exhale, bending at the knees and hinging forward from the hips into a relaxed Forward Bend (see p.162). Place your hands (or fingertips, if less flexible) on the floor.

5 Inhale as you lengthen through the backs of the legs and through the spine, drawing your upper body away from your thighs. Look at the floor slightly ahead of you. ▶

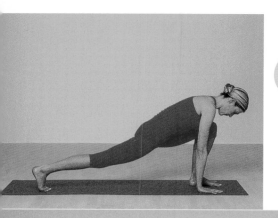

6 Exhale, bending at the knees, and take a large step back with your right foot. Land on the ball of the right foot. Your upper torso is resting on your left thigh. Look down at the floor.

7 Inhale, coming into the basic Lunge Warrior position (see p.166). Extend through the front of the body and look straight ahead.

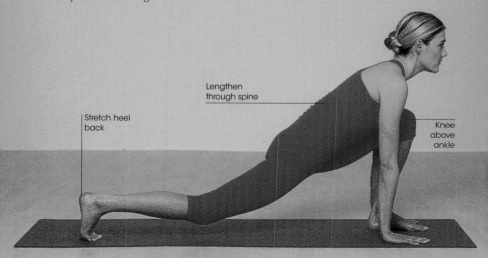

Lengthen through spine

Stretch heel back

Knee above ankle

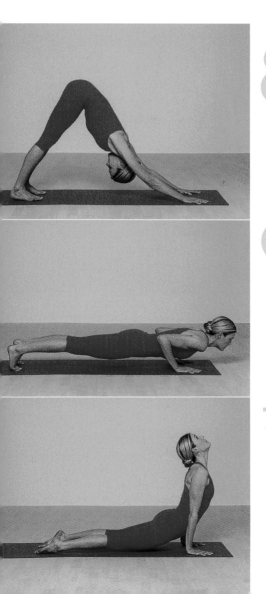

Exhale as you step the left foot back to come into Downward Dog (see p.170). Press your heels toward the floor, but do not force them to the floor. If necessary, keep your knees bent.

Holding the breath out, lower yourself into Crocodile (see p.172). Keep your heels pushing back and your abdomen drawn back toward your spine. (For an alternative way of moving from Step 8 to Step 10, see p.181.)

Inhale as you come into Upward Dog (see p.174). Roll over on to the fronts of your feet, extending through the front of the body and lifting the breastbone. Look up toward the ceiling. ▶

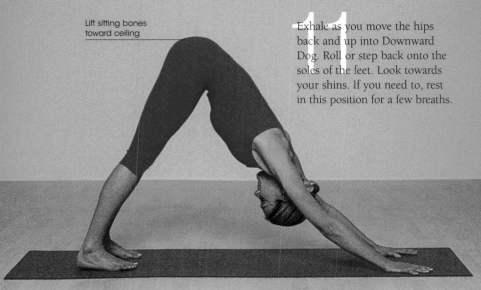

Lift sitting bones
toward ceiling

11 Exhale as you move the hips back and up into Downward Dog. Roll or step back onto the soles of the feet. Look towards your shins. If you need to, rest in this position for a few breaths.

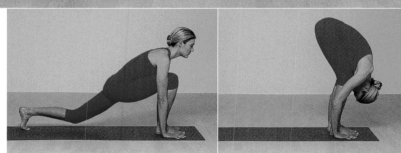

12 Inhale as you step the right foot forward between your hands to move back into Lunge Warrior, coming up onto your fingertips if you need to. If you are very stiff, you may need to take two steps forward.

13 As you exhale, bring your left foot forward to join the right foot and come into an easy Forward Bend, with bent legs if necessary. Relax your shoulders and neck.

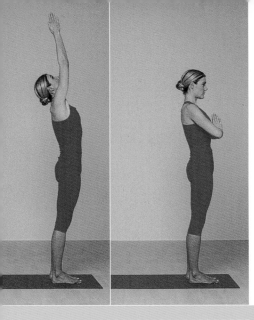

14 Inhale to come up, keeping your knees bent. As you lift up, circle your arms out to the side and bring the palms together above your head, arching the back slightly. Look up at your hands.

15 Exhale as you lower your arms to bring the palms in front of the chest in prayer position. Lower the head to look directly ahead. Repeat the sequence, taking the left leg back at Step 6. This constitutes one round.

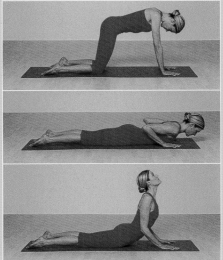

ALTERNATIVE SUB-SEQUENCE

If you find the movements from Step 8 to 10 too strong, try the following more gentle version.

• From Downward Dog, hold the breath out and bring your knees to the floor to come onto all fours.

• Without breathing in, lower yourself to the floor with the hands underneath the shoulders, and the elbows tucked in.

• As you inhale, lift the head and shoulders and extend the top of the chest forward to come into modified Upward Dog with the fronts of the legs on the floor.

triangle

This side-bending posture helps to increase hip-joint flexibility and opens the chest. Feel the energy radiating out from the core of your body. Do not worry if your lower hand is a long way from the floor.

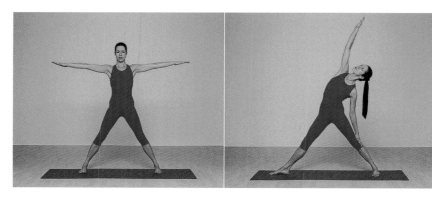

1 Stand with your feet 3 ft (1 m) or more apart, palms together in front of your chest. Look forward. As you breathe in, sweep your arms up and out to the side at shoulder level.

2 Turn your left heel out a little and rotate the right leg out until your toes point to the side. Drop the left arm onto the leg and stretch the right arm up. Take several breaths.

TAKE CARE
• If you have back problems, rest front arm higher up the leg.
• Do not turn your head to look up at your hand if you have neck problems.

3 As you breathe out, reach out sideways over the right leg. At the same time, slide your left hand up to bring the palm against the small of your back. Look along your right arm. Feel your spine lengthen, your chest and hips open to the front.

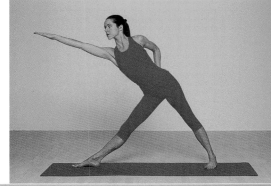

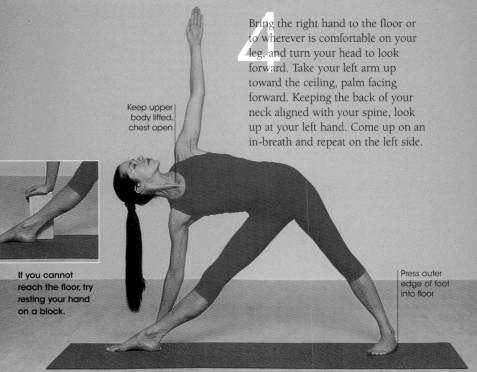

Keep upper body lifted, chest open

4 Bring the right hand to the floor or to wherever is comfortable on your leg, and turn your head to look forward. Take your left arm up toward the ceiling, palm facing forward. Keeping the back of your neck aligned with your spine, look up at your left hand. Come up on an in-breath and repeat on the left side.

If you cannot reach the floor, try resting your hand on a block.

Press outer edge of foot into floor

bent-knee side bend

This sideways-bending posture gives an invigorating stretch through the upper side of the body, while opening the hips and the chest. Keep the back leg strong, and the front hip, knee, and foot in line.

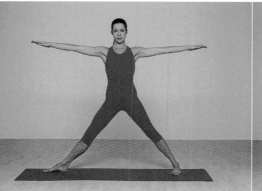 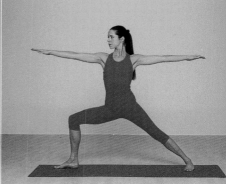

1 Stand with your feet about 3 ft (1 m) or more apart, palms together in front of your chest. As you breathe in, sweep your arms up and out to the sides at shoulder level, palms facing the floor. Turn your left heel out slightly, and rotate the right leg and foot 90 degrees to the right.

2 Breathe in deeply; then, as you exhale, bend the right knee to the side until the knee is above the heel. Turn the upper torso to look along the right arm and feel your tailbone dropping toward the floor. Hold, taking a couple of breaths.

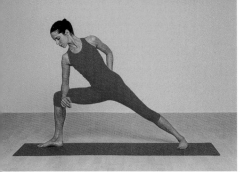

3 On an exhalation, bend to the right, bringing the right forearm to rest on the right thigh. Bring the palm of the left hand on to your sacrum. Open the chest to the front and press the outside edges of the feet to the floor. Look down at your right knee.

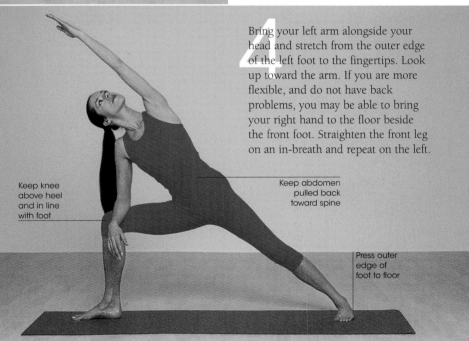

4 Bring your left arm alongside your head and stretch from the outer edge of the left foot to the fingertips. Look up toward the arm. If you are more flexible, and do not have back problems, you may be able to bring your right hand to the floor beside the front foot. Straighten the front leg on an in-breath and repeat on the left.

Keep knee above heel and in line with foot

Keep abdomen pulled back toward spine

Press outer edge of foot to floor

TAKE CARE
• Look straight ahead if you have neck problems. • Keep your forearm on the thigh and your hand on your back if you have HBP.

runner's stretch

Called Runner's Stretch because it works particularly on the hamstrings and calf muscles of the leading leg, this posture also massages and helps tone your digestive organs with every breath.

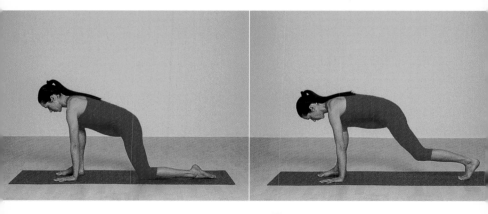

1 Start in the all-fours position, hands shoulder-width apart, fingers spread and pointing forward. Step your right leg forward, bringing the sole of the foot to rest between your hands, so that the knee is directly above the heel. Look down at the floor.

2 Lengthen your upper body forward over the right thigh. Come on to the ball of your left foot and, as you breathe in, lift your left knee away from the floor. Keep the palms of your hands flat on the floor.

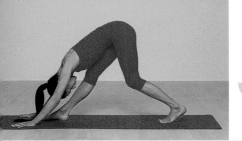

3 As you breathe out, lift the sitting bones up and back, and lengthen through the back of the right leg, keeping the left knee bent.

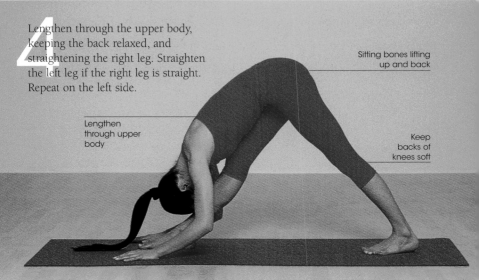

4 Lengthen through the upper body, keeping the back relaxed, and straightening the right leg. Straighten the left leg if the right leg is straight. Repeat on the left side.

Lengthen through upper body

Sitting bones lifting up and back

Keep backs of knees soft

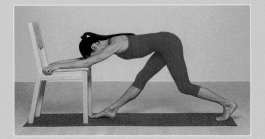

ALTERNATIVE

If you find the stretch too intense, or if you have back problems, HBP, a heart condition, glaucoma, or a detached retina, do the posture using a chair. Hold onto the seat of a chair as you bend forward. If necessary, keep the left leg bent to protect the back.

lunge
twist

This posture combines a twist for the spine with a wide arm stretch to help relieve backaches and stiffness in the shoulders. Focus on breathing smoothly and on broadening across the top of the chest.

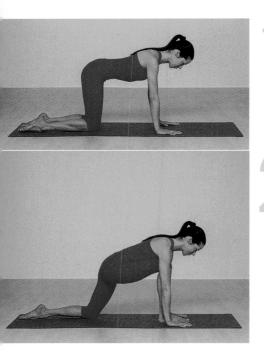

1 Start on your hands and knees, your arms shoulder-width apart. Spread your fingers, with the middle finger pointing directly ahead. Look down at the floor.

2 Bring the right foot forward and place between the hands, so the knee is directly above the ankle and the heels of the hands align with the ankle. Lengthen through the upper body.

TAKE CARE
• Twist cautiously if you have back problems or a hernia.
• If you have neck problems, do not look up.
• Rest the upper hand on the thigh of the bent leg if you have HBP.

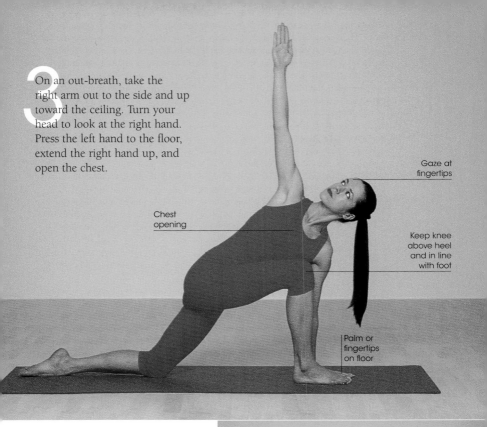

3 On an out-breath, take the right arm out to the side and up toward the ceiling. Turn your head to look at the right hand. Press the left hand to the floor, extend the right hand up, and open the chest.

Gaze at fingertips

Chest opening

Keep knee above heel and in line with foot

Palm or fingertips on floor

4 To come out from the pose, lower your right hand to the floor again and stretch through the back of the right leg. Then come back to the all-fours position. Repeat the sequence on the left side.

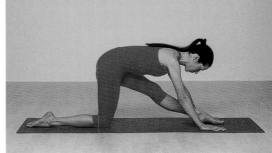

wide leg
forward bend

This posture provides an invigorating stretch to the backs of the legs and inner thighs. It also reverses the effect of gravity on the upper body, easing out the back, and calming the mind.

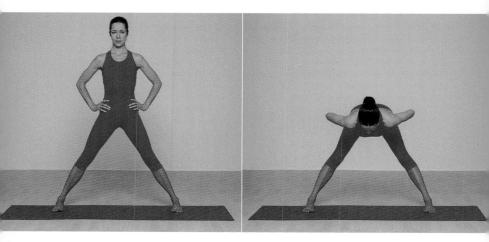

1 Stand with your legs 3 ft (1 m) or so apart, hands on hips, and feet facing forward. Look straight ahead. Draw the muscles in the fronts of the thighs up and out. Lift the breastbone. Breathe in.

2 As you breathe out, hinge forward and down from the hips, keeping the spine long. If you have a back problem, bend your knees before bending forward. Look down.

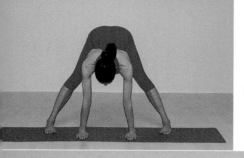

3 Still breathing out, bring your hands to the floor directly below the shoulders. Breathe in, pressing your hands into the floor to lengthen through the arms and back.

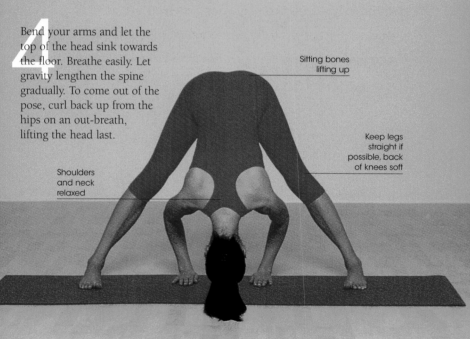

4 Bend your arms and let the top of the head sink towards the floor. Breathe easily. Let gravity lengthen the spine gradually. To come out of the pose, curl back up from the hips on an out-breath, lifting the head last.

Sitting bones lifting up

Keep legs straight if possible, back of knees soft

Shoulders and neck relaxed

TAKE CARE
• If you have back problems, keep the knees bent and/or use a chair for support. • Bend forward halfway, using a chair, if you have HBP, a heart condition, glaucoma, or a detached retina.

side-bending
sequence

This dynamic side-bending sequence can help you feel calm, centered, and invigorated. Try taking three breaths in each stage of the sequence to help the body open and the mind let go.

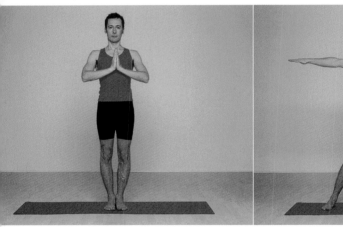

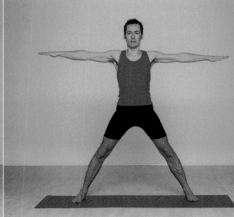

1 Stand with your feet together, hands in prayer position in front of your chest. Standing up tall, take a little time to center yourself, breathing easily and gently pressing the heels of the hands together.

2 Step your feet 3 ft (1 m) or more apart. Then sweep your arms up and out to shoulder level, palms facing down. The arms should feel active, the shoulders relaxed.

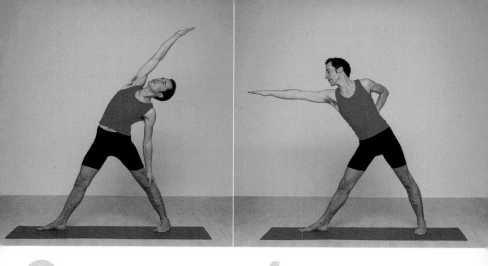

3 Turn the left heel out and rotate the right leg so the toes face the end of the mat. As you breathe in, raise the right arm and arch to the left, opening the right side of the body. Lower the left arm to rest on the left leg.

4 As you breathe out, reach out to the side with the right arm, and bring the left hand onto the lower back. Lengthen through the trunk. Look along the right arm.

5 Bring the right hand onto the right leg, as close to the ankle as you find comfortable. Press the left hand gently against the back to help open the chest. Keep the hips as open as possible. Extend through the spine, with the top of the head moving to the side wall. Look forward. ▶

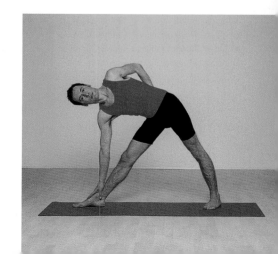

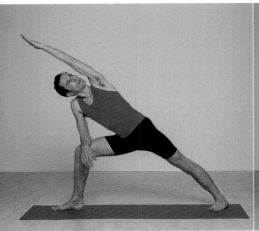

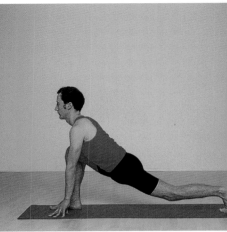

6 Breathing out, bend the right knee over the heel. Bring the right forearm onto the right thigh and rest it there. Stretch the left arm alongside the head. Keep the hips open and turn the head to look up at the arm.

7 On the out-breath, lower your left arm and bring your hands to the floor on each side of, and parallel to, the right foot. Simultaneously, pivot on the ball of your left foot to come into Lunge Warrior (see p.166).

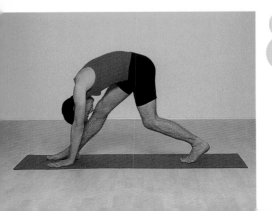

8 Take a step forward with the left foot to come into Runner's Stretch (see p.186). Keeping the left knee bent, stretch through the back of the right leg as much as you find comfortable. Lengthen through your upper body as you fold forward. Visualize your sitting bones moving up and back toward the top of the wall behind you. Keep your back relaxed and your hands on the floor.

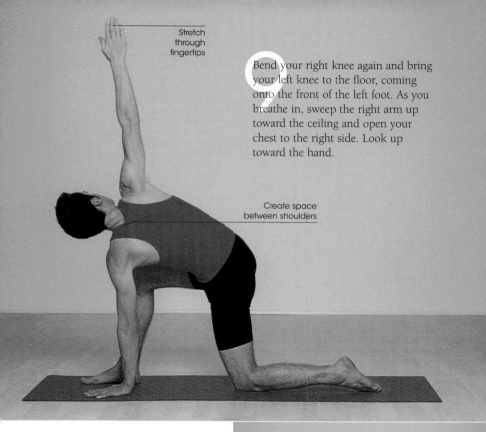

Stretch
through
fingertips

9 Bend your right knee again and bring
your left knee to the floor, coming
onto the front of the left foot. As you
breathe in, sweep the right arm up
toward the ceiling and open your
chest to the right side. Look up
toward the hand.

Create space
between shoulders

10 Bring the right hand back to
the floor on an out-breath. Come
onto the ball of the left foot and
move back into Runner's Stretch.
Remember to lift the sitting bones
up and back while keeping the
upper body soft. ▶

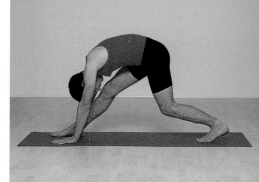

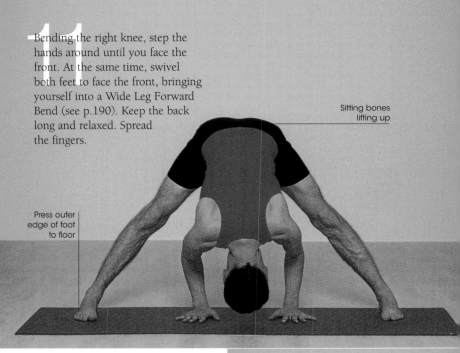

11 Bending the right knee, step the hands around until you face the front. At the same time, swivel both feet to face the front, bringing yourself into a Wide Leg Forward Bend (see p.190). Keep the back long and relaxed. Spread the fingers.

Sitting bones lifting up

Press outer edge of foot to floor

12 Bend your knees and bring your hands onto your hips. As you breathe in, keeping the back relaxed, slowly uncurl your body to come up. Stack the vertebrae up one at a time, finally raising the head to face the front and straightening the legs.

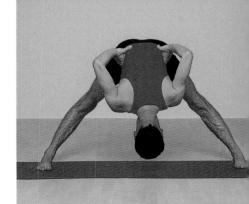

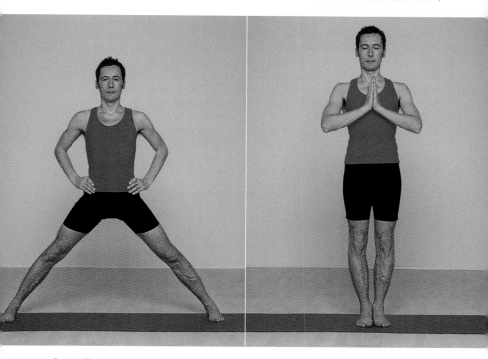

13 Pressing into the outside edges of the feet, rotate the thigh bones out. Press the elbows a little toward the back wall. Open and lift the chest, broadening across the front of the shoulders. Look straight ahead. Take a couple of breaths.

14 Step the feet together, bringing the palms together in front of the chest. Repeat the whole sequence, working on the left side of the body. Then stand quietly with your eyes closed for a short while and experience the energy and the stillness.

child

Child is a restorative pose that gently stretches the spine and postural muscles in the back, while taking your attention inwards. It is a good posture for developing breath awareness.

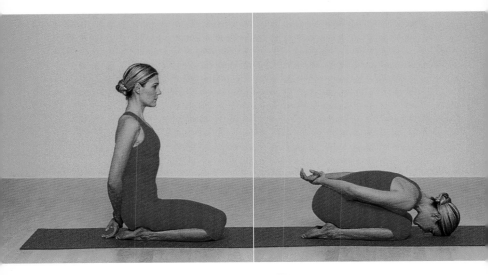

Kneel and sit back on your heels, looking straight ahead. With your hands behind your back, hold one wrist with the other hand. Lengthen through the spine. Breathe in.

As you exhale, fold forward over the knees, hinging from the hips. Bring your forehead to the floor. (Rest your forehead on a block or other support if this is difficult.)

3 Bring your arms to the floor alongside the body, or, as shown, beside the head. Rest in the pose, focusing on breathing quietly and steadily. Child can also be done dynamically (if you do not suffer from epilepsy), moving alternately between Step 1 and 2 with the breath five to 10 times.

Be aware of breath in back ribs

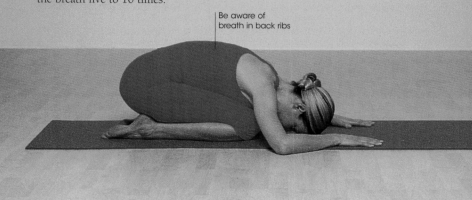

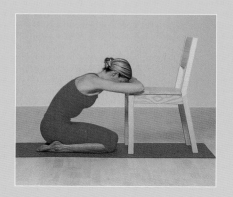

ALTERNATIVE

If you have back problems, HBP, glaucoma, or a detached retina, do not bring the head to the floor. Instead, rest your head on your hands with your forearms on the seat of a chair.

hare

Like Child, Hare is a restorative pose; it stretches the spine and helps relieve stiffness in the shoulder girdle. Try to let the spine lengthen and the shoulders relax on the out-breath.

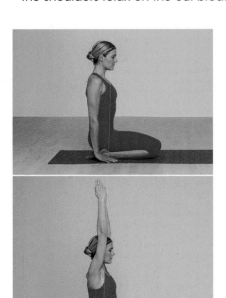

1 Sit up straight, sitting back on your heels. Press your hands into the mat on each side of your torso, fingers pointing forward. Lengthen through the spine and look straight ahead.

2 On an in-breath, circle your arms out to the sides of your body and up above your head. Lower them on the out-breath, and raise them again on the in-breath.

TAKE CARE
If you have back problems, glaucoma, or a detached retina, stretch forward with your hands on a chair.

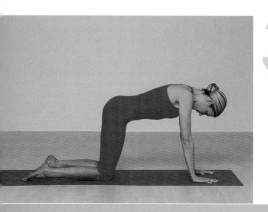

3 As you exhale, lower your arms forward to come onto your hands and knees. Your hands should be shoulder-width apart and your knees under your hips.

4 On an exhalation, keeping your hands still, take your hips back to sit on your heels. Feel the stretch through the shoulders and the back, creeping the hands forward to increase the stretch. Take several deep, slow breaths. Relax the arms and sit back up on an in-breath.

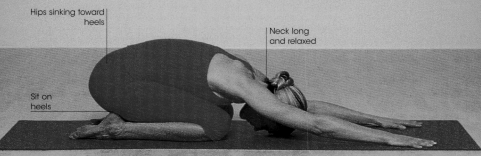

Hips sinking toward heels

Neck long and relaxed

Sit on heels

camel

Feel the energy surge through your upper body in this invigorating, back-bending posture. Lift up through the front of the body and let the tailbone drop as you arch back, to create space in the spine.

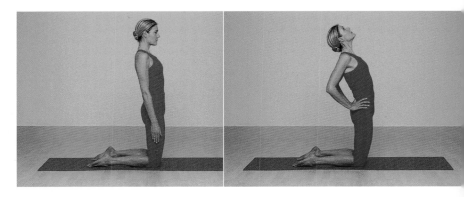

1 Kneel with the body upright and the legs hip-width apart. Press the hands against the thighs, tuck the tailbone under, and draw the abdomen in. Lift the breastbone, relax the shoulders.

2 Place your hands on your hips. As you breathe in, lift the chest, take the elbows back, and look up toward the ceiling. Exhale and hold the position as you continue to breathe steadily.

TAKE CARE
• Be very cautious going beyond Step 2 if you have back problems, a hernia, recent abdominal surgery, HBP, or heart disease.
• If you have neck problems, do not take your head back at Step 4.

3 As you breathe in, circle your right arm forward and up beside your head, and as you exhale, circle it back down to your right heel. Repeat with the left arm.

4 Keeping the thighs perpendicular, lengthen the front of the body as you slowly arch back to touch your heels. Hold for three to five breaths. Breathe in, release the hands, and come back up to kneeling upright.

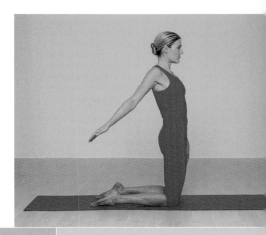

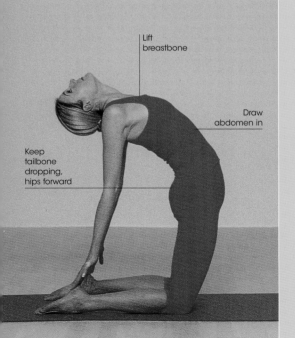

Lift breastbone

Draw abdomen in

Keep tailbone dropping, hips forward

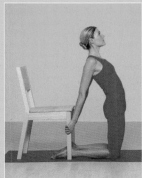

ALTERNATIVE

If your body is stiff, do not try to bring your arms right down to your heels. Instead, position a chair over your feet and lean back to hold onto its legs as far down as is comfortable.

shoulder stand
against a wall

A rejuvenating posture that reverses the effects of gravity on the body and stimulates the brain's balance centers. You may need to use a blanket under the shoulders (see p.208) to keep the neck free.

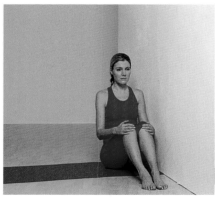

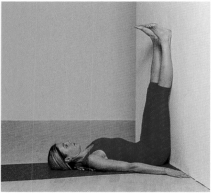

1 Sit up straight alongside a wall with your knees bent and your left hip against the wall. Take several breaths to centre yourself.

2 Swivel around, supporting yourself with your hands, to lie on your back with your buttocks against the wall and your legs up the wall. Draw your shoulders away from your ears.

TAKE CARE

• Stop at Step 2 if you are seriously overweight or menstruating, or have neck problems, HBP, a heart condition, or a detached retina.

• If you have back problems, lie with your knees bent over a chair.

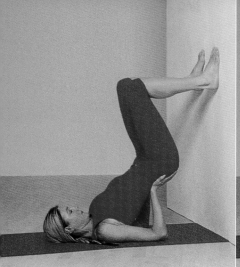

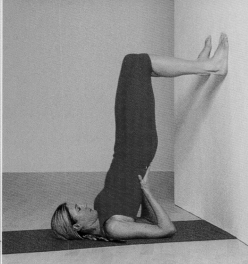

3 Bend your knees to bring the soles of the feet against the wall. Breathe in and push against the wall to lift your bottom off the floor. Support your back with your hands.

4 Keep pushing against the wall to lengthen through the front of the body until your back and thighs are perpendicular. If you feel any discomfort in the neck, come down and seek advice before trying again.

5 Make sure you are breathing easily. Lift the left leg away from the wall and point the foot straight up to the ceiling. Bring it back to the wall and do the same with the right leg. ▶

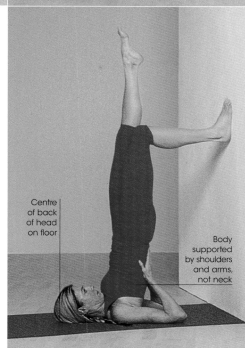

Centre of back of head on floor

Body supported by shoulders and arms, not neck

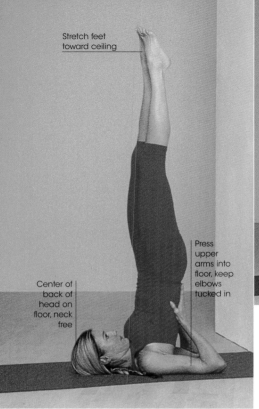

Stretch feet toward ceiling

Press upper arms into floor, keep elbows tucked in

Center of back of head on floor, neck free

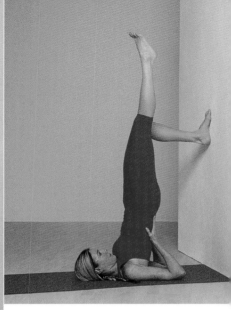

7 To come out of the pose, bend your left knee to bring the sole of your left foot back to the wall. Keep stretching up through the spine. Continue to support your back with your hands.

6 Bring one leg and then the other away from the wall to come into a Full Shoulder Stand. Slide your hands closer to your shoulders to help keep the body upright. Hold for about 30 seconds to start with, increasing the time as you become more familiar with the pose. Breathe normally, stretching the feet toward the ceiling and lengthening through the body.

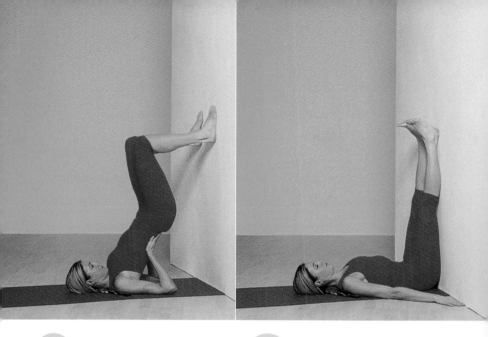

8 Bend your right knee to bring your right foot to the wall. Breathing normally, start to lower your spine to the floor, keeping the back supported as you come down.

9 When your lower back is on the floor, take your arms out to the side and stay in the position for a few breaths with your legs stretched up the wall.

10 On an out-breath, roll over onto your right side with your knees bent. Stay there for a short while, breathing easily. Try Easy Fish (see p.212) before moving on to practice any other postures.

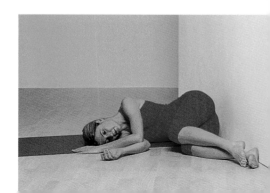

full shoulder stand

If you find Shoulder Stand Against a Wall easy, try the full version. In the final position, focus on lifting up through the spine and stretching the legs up. Keep relaxed and breathe smoothly and deeply.

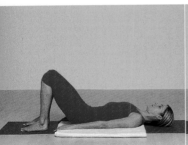 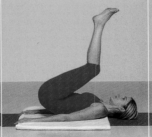 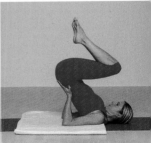

1 Lie on a folded blanket with your knees bent and your arms by your side, palms facing down. The back of the head and neck should be off the blanket.

2 On an inhalation, bend your knees over your chest and swing the legs up. Press strongly into the floor with your hands and forearms.

3 Bring your hands up to support your back, keeping your upper arms on the floor. Press your hands into the back to bring your weight onto the tops of your shoulders, making sure your neck is free and relaxed.

TAKE CARE

• As for Shoulder Stand Against a Wall. • When using a blanket, make sure the tops of the shoulders line up with the edge of the blanket and the neck is off the blanket and free.

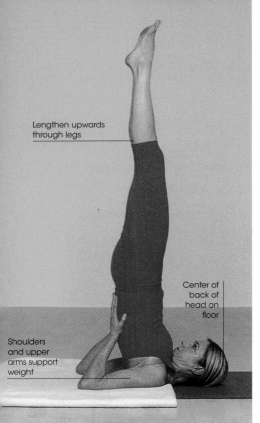

Lengthen upwards
through legs

Center of
back of
head on
floor

Shoulders
and upper
arms support
weight

4 Pushing your upper arms and elbows into the floor, slide your hands toward your shoulders to bring your upper body vertical. Slowly straighten your legs toward the ceiling and bring the elbows closer together. Breathe easily. Stay only for a short time to begin with.

5 On an exhalation, bend the knees toward the head and roll down, supporting the back with the hands. You may need to let your head and shoulders come off the floor as you roll down.

6 Come into a relaxed sitting Forward Bend with knees bent, as shown here, or simply lie on your back with your knees bent for a few breaths.

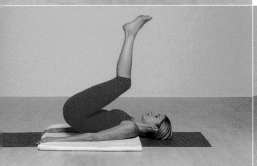

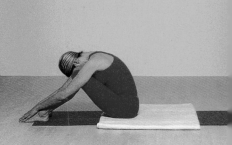

plow

A soothing pose, Plow combines some of the benefits of an inversion with a strong stretch through the upper back and the back of the legs. Avoid altogether if you have neck problems.

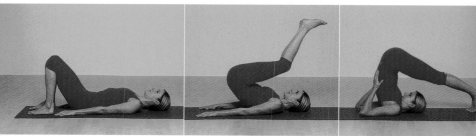

1 Lie on your back with your knees bent, feet hip-width apart. Place your arms beside your body, palms facing down. Take several breaths.

2 On an inhalation, bend the knees over the chest and swing the legs up. Press strongly into the ground with your hands and forearms.

3 Bring your hands up to support your back, keeping your upper arms on the floor as for Full Shoulder Stand (see p.208). Bring your weight onto the tops of your shoulders, making sure your neck is free and relaxed. Stretch your legs back and bring your feet to the floor.

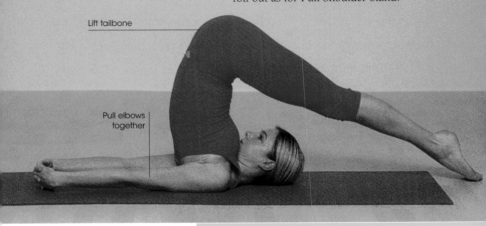

Lengthen up through your spine and stretch your arms out along the floor behind you with the fingers interlocked. Stay in the pose for a short while to begin with, breathing quietly. Then bend the legs again and, supporting your back, roll out as for Full Shoulder Stand.

Lift tailbone

Pull elbows together

TAKE CARE

• If you are seriously overweight, or are menstruating, have HBP, a heart condition, or a detached retina, stop at Step 3; relax and breathe easily.
• Lie on your back with knees bent over a chair if you have back problems.

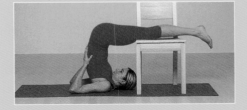

ALTERNATIVE

If you cannot reach the floor with your feet, bend your knees toward your forehead or practice with your thighs resting on a chair, as shown. Support your back with your hands.

easy fish

This posture provides an excellent counterstretch for the back and the neck after doing the Full Shoulder Stand (see p.208). Easy Fish stretches the front of the body, opens the chest, extends the spine, and strengthens the upper arms.

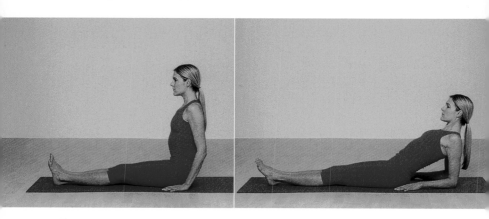

1 Sit up straight with your legs stretched out in front of you, feet together. Place your arms down by your sides. Look straight ahead. Push into the hands to lengthen through the upper body.

2 Lean back on your forearms with your elbows positioned underneath your shoulders, fingers pointing forward. Keep looking straight ahead.

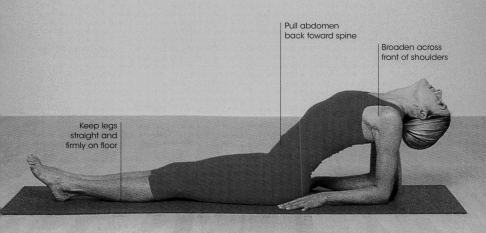

Pull abdomen
back toward spine

Broaden across
front of shoulders

Keep legs
straight and
firmly on floor

3 Stretch your toes away. Breathing in, press your forearms down and open your chest toward the ceiling. Slowly take your head back to look up at the ceiling, arching your back gently. Breathe deeply into the chest.

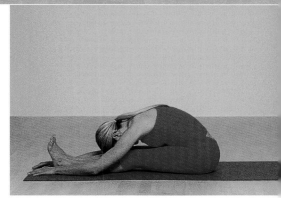

TAKE CARE
• Keep the head in line with your spine if you have neck problems.
• Do not arch the back excessively if you have back problems.

4 To come out of the pose, bring your head forward, then press into the forearms and hands to sit up. Fold forward, resting your forehead on your knees. If you need to, bend your knees.

sitting
forward stretch

This energy-balancing posture encourages flexibility in the spine and stretches the hamstrings, while allowing the mind to settle on your inner awareness as you relax forwards.

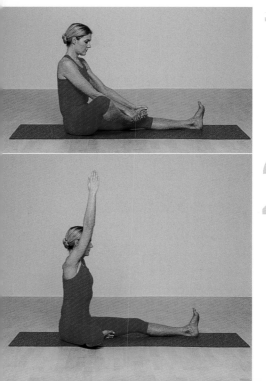

1 Sit with your feet stretched out in front of you. Press your hands into the floor at the sides of your hips to bring yourself onto your sitting bones. Then bring the sole of your right foot onto the inside of your left thigh, close to the groin.

2 Allow the right knee to sink to the floor. Bring your right hip forward to align yourself with your left leg. If your knee is a long way off the floor, support it with a pillow. As you breathe in, bring your arms up beside your head. Look straight ahead.

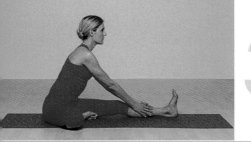

As you breathe out, hinge forward from the hips. Keep the back long and your gaze straight ahead. Bring your hands onto your leg. Breathe in, lengthening through the spine.

As you breathe out, lengthen forward again and, if you are able to, hold on to your left foot. Bend the elbows to gently bring the upper body closer to the leg without straining the back. Relax, breathing easily. Sit up slowly on an in-breath and repeat on the other side.

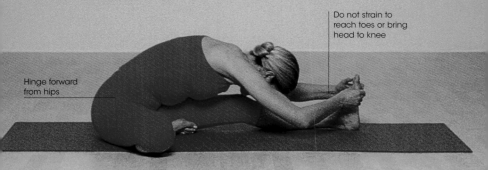

Do not strain to reach toes or bring head to knee

Hinge forward from hips

ALTERNATIVE

If you have tight hamstrings, inflexible hips or back, or a hernia, try sitting on a block, or place a folded blanket under the bent leg as you reach forward. If necessary, hold onto a belt that is looped around the foot, to avoid straining your back.

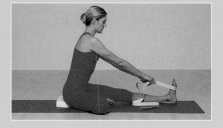

supine
butterfly

This relaxing posture can help release tension in the abdomen and pelvic area, and relieve period pains. The benefits are enhanced by practicing Abdominal Breathing (see p.225) in the pose.

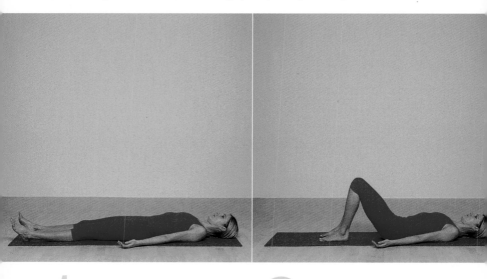

1 Lie on your back with your legs stretched out and your arms away to the sides of the body, the backs of the hands on the floor. Lengthen through the back of your neck.

2 Bend your knees, sliding your feet close to your buttocks. Feel yourself broadening across the top of the chest as you draw the shoulders down away from the ears.

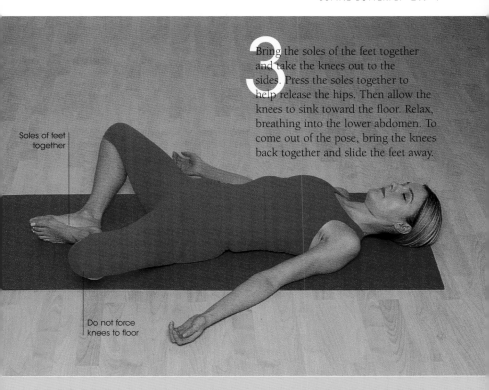

3 Bring the soles of the feet together and take the knees out to the sides. Press the soles together to help release the hips. Then allow the knees to sink toward the floor. Relax, breathing into the lower abdomen. To come out of the pose, bring the knees back together and slide the feet away.

Soles of feet together

Do not force knees to floor

ALTERNATIVE

Do not try to force the knees to the floor. If your knees do not reach the floor, or if you suffer from sacroiliac back pain, support the legs with pillows or folded blankets. To focus on Abdominal Breathing, try placing your hands on the abdomen.

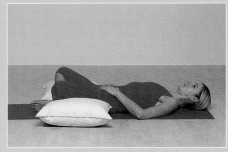

kneeling stretch
sequence

This is a calming sequence that helps you unwind and balance your energy. It is especially beneficial at the end of a stressful day, when it will refresh your mind and body, enabling you to enjoy the evening.

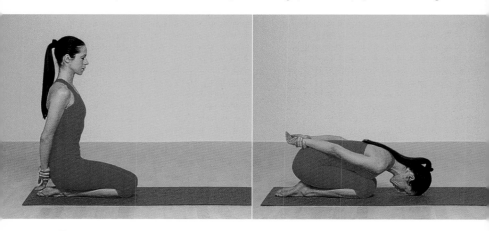

1 Sit back on your heels and hold on to your right wrist with your left hand. Lengthening through the spine and back of the neck, look straight ahead. Take several breaths with your eyes closed to center yourself. Breathe in.

2 As you breathe out, fold forward to bring the upper body on to the thighs. Breathe in and come back up to sitting. Then, as you breathe out, fold forward again.

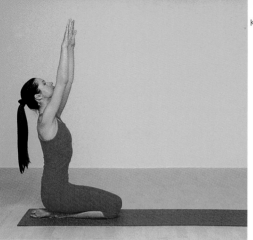

Breathing in, sit up. At the same time, circle your arms out to the side and up above your head. Look up at your fingertips.

Keeping your arms raised, fold forward on the out-breath. With your arms out in front, in line with your shoulders, gently stretch through the spine.

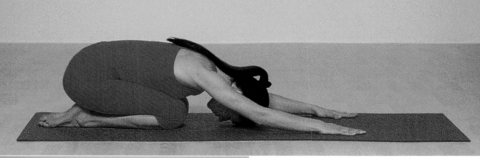

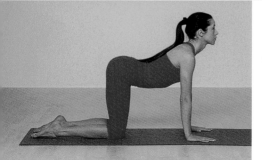

As you breathe in, come up onto all fours. Make sure your legs are hip-width apart and your wrists in line with your shoulders. Breathe out, then breathe in and tilt the tailbone up, taking the top of the chest forward as you look directly to the front. ▶

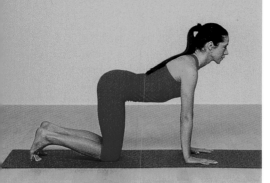

6 Breathe out. Then, as you breathe in, tuck your toes under. Make sure the insides of your elbows are facing each other, your hands are parallel, and your fingers point forward. Look straight ahead.

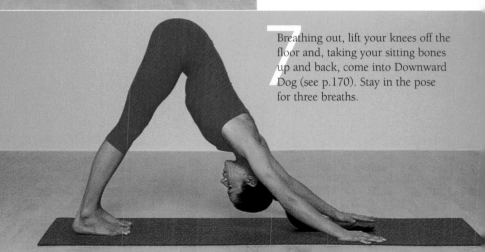

7 Breathing out, lift your knees off the floor and, taking your sitting bones up and back, come into Downward Dog (see p.170). Stay in the pose for three breaths.

8 Breathing out, come down into an all-fours position again. Lengthen through the arms and keep the shoulders down away from the ears. Look down at the floor. Breathe in and come onto the front of the feet.

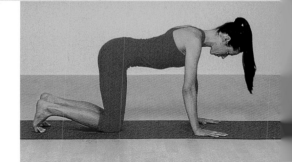

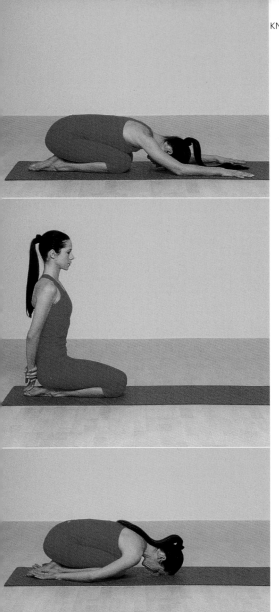

9 Keeping your hands still, take the hips back to sit on your heels as you breathe out. Stretch through the spine and relax the forearms to the floor.

10 On the in-breath, sit up, keeping the back straight. Bring your arms behind you, and hold your right wrist with your left hand. Lift though the spine and the front of the body, broadening across the top of the chest.

11 Breathing out, fold forward over the thighs to bring the forehead to the floor. Bring your arms down by your sides, palms up. Relax in this position, breathing quietly, for one or two minutes before sitting up.

sitting twist

This simple spinal twist encourages spinal flexibility, helps relieve stiffness in the shoulders and neck, and stretches respiratory muscles. Close your eyes and focus awareness on sensations within the body.

1 Sit up straight with your feet stretched out in front of you. Pressing down with your hands, make sure you are sitting toward the front edge of your sitting bones. If you have tight hamstrings, sit on a block.

2 Draw your right foot up beside your left knee and place it on the outside of the left knee. Clasp the shin with both hands and pull against it to lengthen through the spine and the front of the body.

TAKE CARE

Twist with caution if you have back problems, or a hernia, or have had recent abdominal surgery.

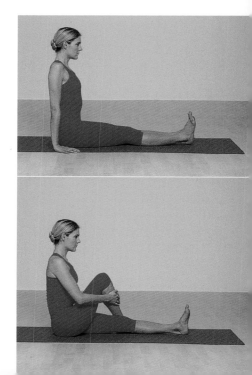

3 Take your right hand to the floor behind you and hook your left arm around your right knee. Facing forward, breathe in as you lengthen through the upper body.

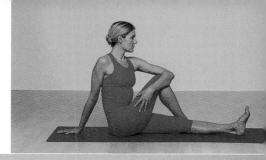

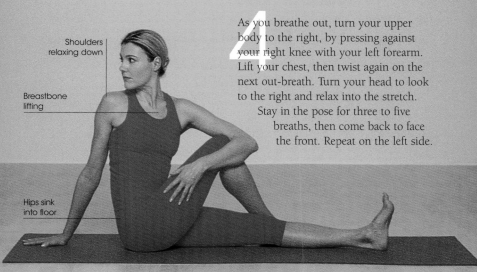

Shoulders relaxing down

Breastbone lifting

Hips sink into floor

4 As you breathe out, turn your upper body to the right, by pressing against your right knee with your left forearm. Lift your chest, then twist again on the next out-breath. Turn your head to look to the right and relax into the stretch. Stay in the pose for three to five breaths, then come back to face the front. Repeat on the left side.

5 If you are more flexible, you may find it more effective to bring the back of the left arm onto the outside of the right knee. As you breathe out, keep the arm straight and pressing against the leg. Stretch the fingertips toward the floor to turn to the side.

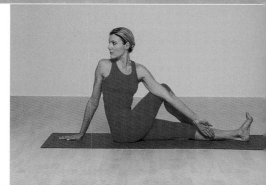

breathing
practices

The following breathing practices can be done simply to improve your awareness of the breath, but they are also particularly useful in helping to quiet the mind for meditation (see p.230).

The breathing practices described on the following six pages will help improve your breath awareness and encourage calmness and mental clarity. They are generally practiced after doing some yoga postures or some simple stretching. They help loosen up the body, so that it is easier for you to be relaxed during the breathing practices.

The practices of Mock Inhalation (see p.226) and Forced Exhalation (see p.228) are best learned with a teacher. If you have any problems, be sure to seek help.

Audible breath

A simple practice, audible breath helps make the breath smooth and even. It calms and centers the mind, and helps you to let go of tension. It can be practiced for its own sake and also during posture work, to help you remain focused.

To begin the practice, breathe through the mouth. Slightly closing the throat, make a gentle sighing "Ahhhh" sound as you breathe in and a sighing "Haaaa" sound as you breathe out.

When you have gotten a feel for this, try to achieve the same sound in the throat while breathing with your mouth closed. It may help to imagine that you are breathing through a hole in the front of the throat. Breathe smoothly and evenly, and keep your awareness on the breath. The sound of the breath can be quite subtle; only you need to hear it.

supine abdominal breathing

This practice relaxes the body and the mind, and is good for letting go of tension. Be aware of how easily the breath flows, and of the feeling of calm alertness in the mind at the end of the practice.

1 Lie on your back with your knees bent, feet about hip-width apart. Allow your breath to settle into a smooth, natural rhythm. Then become aware of the rise and fall of the abdomen as you breathe in and out. Focus on the out-breath and very gradually allow it to become longer than the in-breath.

2 Make the out-breath slower and more complete by drawing the abdomen back toward the spine as you exhale. Relax as you breathe in, allowing the abdomen to swell out. Breathe like this for a while.

3 Emphasize the out-breath more by drawing up the pelvic floor muscles (as if stopping yourself from urinating). Now, as you breathe in, keep the abdomen and pelvic floor gently contracted. Feel the breath in the ribcage. As you exhale, emphasize the contraction. After a while, relax and let the breath return to normal.

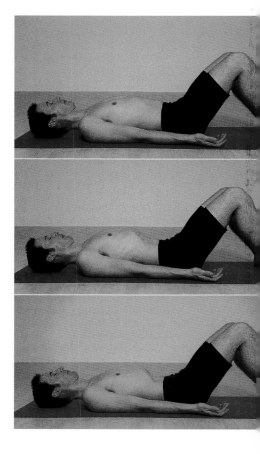

mock inhalation

This practice increases awareness of the diaphragm in breathing and increases its strength and flexibility. It involves taking a full exhalation, and then closing the throat (as if you were holding your breath) and expanding the ribs as if breathing in – a "mock inhalation."

You can do mock inhalation lying on your back (see right) or standing (see below). Do three rounds of the practice, following the instructions detailed at right carefully. Breathe normally for about 20 seconds between each round. After you have completed the practice, feel the quality of the breath. If your first normal in-breath is rushed, practice mock inhalation more gently.

TAKE CARE

• Avoid if you have HBP or active inflammation or bleeding in the abdominal region.
• This practice is best avoided during menstruation, as it creates strong negative pressures in the abdomen.

ALTERNATIVE

Stand with your legs about hip-width apart, your knees slightly bent. Lean forward a little way, rounding your back slightly. Rest your hands lightly on your thighs, your elbows slightly out to the side. Follow Steps 2 and 3 shown at right.

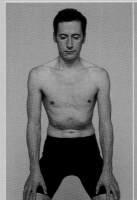
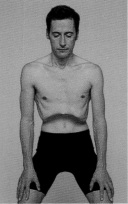

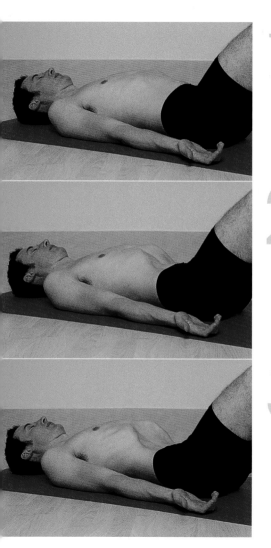

1 Lie on the floor with your knees bent, arms away from the side of the body, palms up. Allow the breath to settle into a natural, regular rhythm.

2 Breathe in deeply, allowing the abdomen to swell out. Then breathe out completely, drawing the abdomen back toward the spine at the same time.

3 Relax the abdomen, close the throat, and simultaneously expand the chest, without breathing in, to suck the abdomen up under the ribcage. Hold until you need to breathe in. To breathe in, relax the ribs first, open the throat, and, contracting the abdominal muscles slightly, let the breath flow in, in a slow, controlled way.

forced exhalation

This practice involves a forced exhalation and a passive in-breath. The intense focus on the out-breath helps clear the mind of distractions and balance the nervous system.

Do three rounds, following the instructions at right carefully, and breathing naturally for about 20 seconds between each rounds. Maintain the same number of exhalations in each round. At the end of the third round, exhale completely and allow a short, natural pause with the breath held out. The next in-breath should be smooth and unhurried. Sit quietly, let the breath be free, and be aware of the smoothness and quietness of the breath and the mind.

During the practice, maintain a steady, even rhythm – slow down if necessary. Never try to keep going if you get out of breath. As you become more familiar with the practice, you can increase the number of exhalations per round.

BLOWING OUT THE CANDLE

This preliminary practice will help you get the feel for the correct action of the abdomen in Forced Exhalation. Rest your right hand on the abdomen and bring your left hand in front of you. Imagine that there is a candle in front of your left hand. Take half a breath in and try to blow it out. Feel the abdomen sharply contract away from your hand and then automatically relax back toward it.

Repeatedly try to blow out the candle. Then try with the mouth closed, by exhaling sharply through the nostrils.

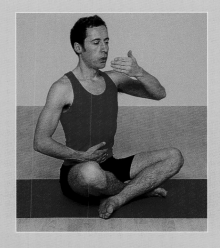

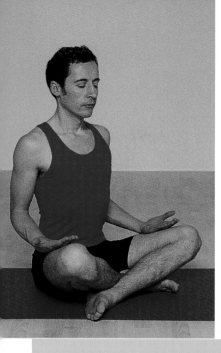

1 Sit cross-legged, spine and head erect, with your hands resting on your thighs, palms facing up. Close your eyes. Let the breath settle into a regular rhythm, emphasizing the out-breath.

2 Breathe in halfway and then exhale forcibly by sharply pulling the abdomen in. Immediately allow the abdomen to relax, so the in-breath is effortless and completely passive.

3 Repeatedly exhale, forcibly in this way up to a maximum of 10 times. This constitutes one round. Then breathe normally for 20 seconds.

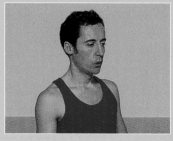

ALTERNATIVE

Sit or stand. Take a full breath in. Breathe out through the mouth in short, rapid puffs, with a brief pause between each puff, until the lungs are empty. Close your mouth and allow a natural pause with the breath held out. Then breathe in slowly and smoothly.

TAKE CARE

• If you become dizzy or breathless during the practice, stop, take a break, then try more slowly and less forcefully.
• If both nostrils are congested, you are menstruating, you have HBP, or you suffer from epilepsy, do the alternative, above.

meditation

Meditation involves silencing the mind and realizing the vital energy that constitutes the core of our being. Regular meditation has great restorative powers, helping to bring your energies into balance.

We cannot meditate by seeking to shut out the world around us or by completely ignoring our senses, thoughts, or emotions. But we can progressively let go of them, so that they do not cloud our consciousness, our awareness.

Sit comfortably in a basic sitting position (see p.141) with your head, neck, and spine erect. If you are more flexible, sit as shown opposite, with your thumb and index finger together in the mudra symbolizing the link between individual and universal energy. Be aware of your surroundings. Close your eyes and be aware of sounds and other sensations, like the touch of the air on your skin. Let the world be there without reacting to it. Become aware of your body. As you breathe out, let go of tension – in your face, your neck, your shoulders, your arms, and your legs. Be aware of your breath, which is your constant connection with the world around you. Be aware of the breath in the nostrils as you breathe in and out. Be aware of it passing through the nostrils and down

PRACTICAL MATTERS

• Choose a time when you can remain undisturbed for at least 15 minutes.
• Choose a room (or outdoor space) that is quiet, uncluttered, and not cold.
• Choose a posture – sitting or kneeling on the floor or sitting in a chair – that you will be able to sustain easily for some time.

the back of the throat to the chest as you breathe in. Feel it rising up from the chest through the back of the throat and out through the nostrils as you breathe out.

Then become aware of the space inside your head, your throat, and your neck. Be aware of the space in the right side of the chest, in the left side. Be aware of the space in the right shoulder, right arm, right hand; in the left shoulder, left arm, left hand; the space in the right hip, right leg, right foot; in the left hip, left leg, left foot. Be aware of the space above and below the navel, at the base of the spine, and in the pelvis.

Be aware of the space in the whole body. Be aware of space around the body, and the infinite space beyond. Be aware of yourself as a center of consciousness – with no separation between inside and outside. Stay with this awareness. Slowly become aware once more of your breath, your body, your surroundings.

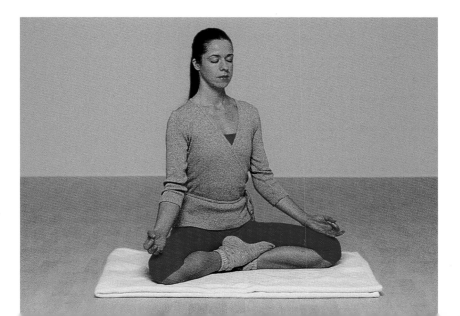

relaxation

At the end of your yoga session, stay quiet for a while to reinforce the restorative and regenerative benefits. This simple relaxation practice will take about 15 to 20 minutes. Make sure you are warm enough.

Lie on the floor, with your knees bent and your arms away from the body. Become aware of your body and how it feels. Lift your hips slightly and extend your tailbone toward your feet, and then lower the hips again, easing out the lower back. Slide your feet along the floor to stretch your legs out (unless this incurs lower back pain, in which case keep your knees bent).

Allow the legs and feet to roll outward. Tuck in your chin and then release it to bring the center of the back of your head onto the floor. If your neck feels uncomfortable like this, try resting it on a pillow or folded blanket.

Now relax your body part by part, starting with your toes and ending with your head. There is no need to do anything active, just take your attention to each part of the body in turn: feet, legs, hips, hands, arms, shoulders, torso, neck, head. Close your eyes and mouth. Be still.

Bring your attention to your breath and let it settle into a natural, regular rhythm. Do not try to breathe in any particular way; simply observe the movement of the breath in and out of the body. As you breathe in, the abdomen gently rises and as you breathe out, it sinks back down again. Gradually allow the out-breath to become a little longer than the in-breath, and be aware that as you breathe out, the body becomes a little more relaxed, a little heavier, seeming to sink into the floor.

Keeping your focus on the breath, count your breaths up to 20 and then back down again. One is an in-breath, two an out-breath, and so on. On the way down from 20, when you reach 10, only count your out-breaths until you reach zero. If you are distracted by thoughts, sounds, or other sensations, return to the breath and the counting.

When you reach zero, let go of the focus on the breath and be aware of the space in front of your eyes; the stillness and the silence. Notice how quiet the breath is, how quiet the mind is. Everything you hear and feel is taking place within your consciousness – you are aware of everything, but there is no need to focus on anything. You are wholly in the present moment – just being. Enjoy this feeling of peace and quiet for as long as it lasts.

Become aware of your body again, the floor beneath you, and the walls around you. Be aware of sounds outside and inside the room. Wriggle your toes and fingers, your hands and your feet. Take one or two deep breaths to bring more energy into the body, and then stretch your arms over your head and give a long sigh. Turn onto your right side and stay there with your eyes closed for a few moments, and then slowly sit up and open your eyes.

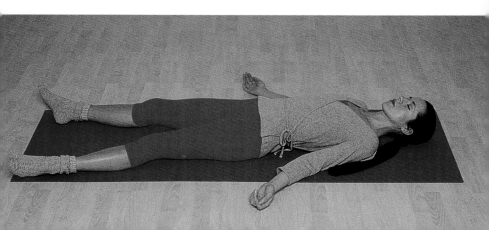

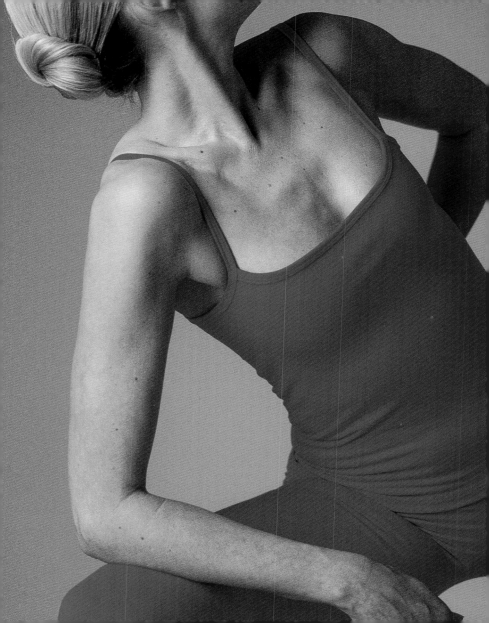

programs

Here are seven programs for those times in the day when you need a quick lift. Remember to take time to center yourself before doing them and time to absorb their effects afterward. Their benefits will be greatly enhanced if you remember that yoga is also about lifestyle and attitude.

① start the
day right

Liven yourself up before breakfast with Sectional Breathing (see p.149) or Mock Inhalation (see p.226), some breathe-and-stretch exercises (see p.150), followed by these postures. For a more dynamic start to the day, do the Sun Salute (see p.176) before the postures. Early morning is also a good time for Meditation (see p.230).

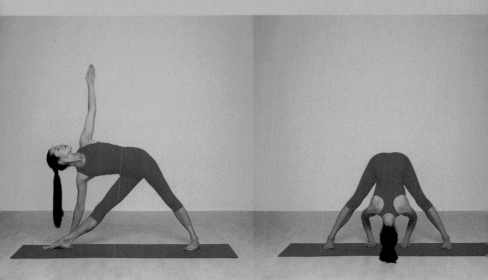

① Triangle (see pp.182–183)

② Wide Leg Forward Bend (pp.190–191)

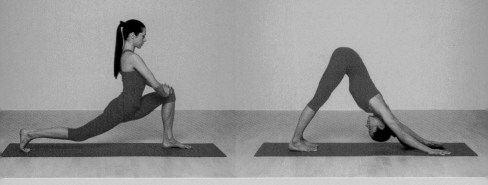

3 Lunge Warrior (see pp.166–169)

4 Downward Dog (see pp.170–171)

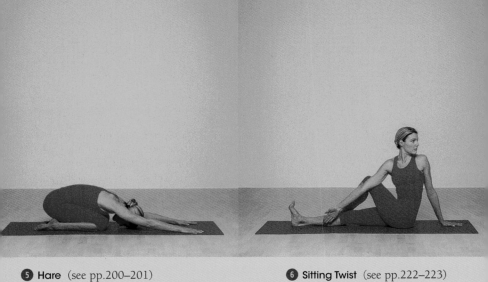

5 Hare (see pp.200–201)

6 Sitting Twist (see pp.222–223)

2 midmorning
boost

Instead of grabbing a coffee, cigarette, or cookie, try these postures. In the workplace you may be able to find a quiet space to do them. If not, some breathe-and-stretch exercises (see p.150) can be done at your desk. If time is really short, Audible Breath (see p.224) or Forced Exhalation (see p.228) will leave you energized, your mind clear.

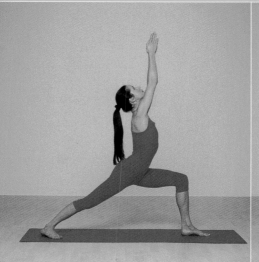

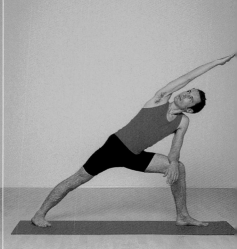

1 Warrior (see pp.164–165)

2 Bent-Knee Side Bend (pp.184–185)

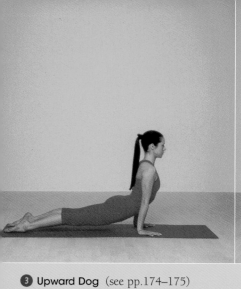

3 **Upward Dog** (see pp.174–175)

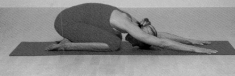

4 **Hare** (see pp.200–201)

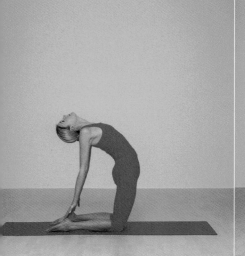

5 **Camel** (see pp.202–203)

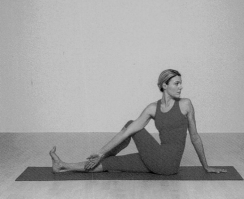

6 **Sitting Twist** (see pp.222–223)

(3) evening recharge

After a hard day at work or a long day with the children, stretch out those tired muscles and stiff joints with these postures. Do some breathe-and-stretch exercises (see p.150) first, and practice Abdominal Breathing (see p.225) while in Supine Butterfly (see p.216), then relax. Early evening is also a good time to practice Meditation (see p.230).

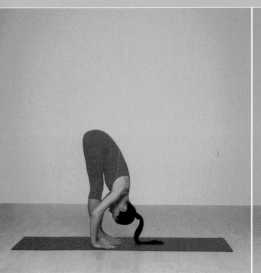

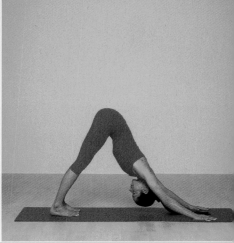

① **Forward Bend** (see pp.162–163)

② **Downward Dog** (see pp.170–171)

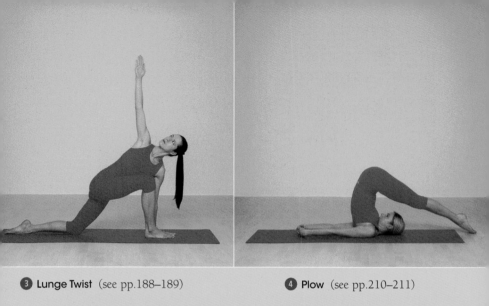

3 Lunge Twist (see pp.188–189)

4 Plow (see pp.210–211)

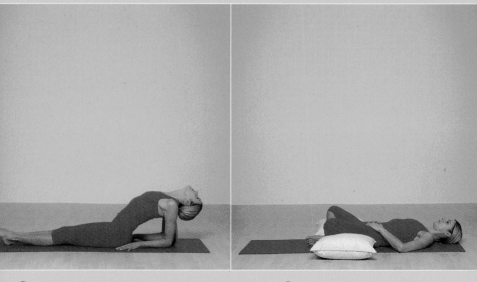

5 Easy Fish (see pp.212–213)

6 Supine Butterfly (see pp.216–217)

4 prepare for the
next day

Here is a routine to stretch the body gently and counter the pull of gravity just before going to bed. In bed, do Abdominal Breathing (see p.225) first, then relax, repeating the following affirmation: *"My energy is strong"* (with palms on abdomen, then on ribcage, then fingers on top of breastbone); *"I am ready for life"* (arms out to side).

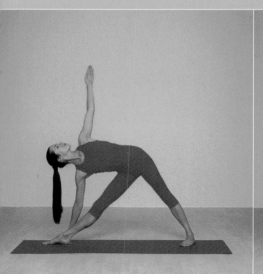

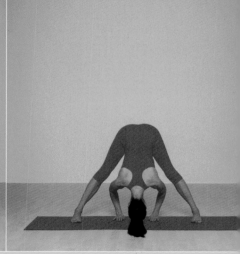

1 Triangle (see pp.182–183)

2 Wide Leg Forward Bend (pp.190–19)

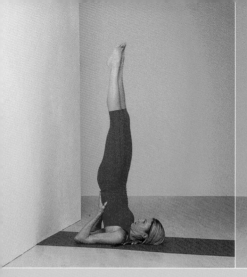

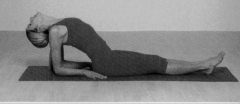

3 Shoulder Stand Against a Wall (pp.204–207)

4 Easy Fish (see pp.212–213)

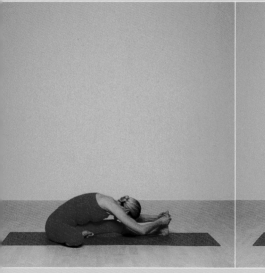

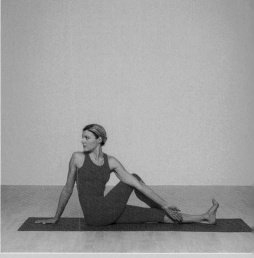

5 Sitting Forward Stretch (see pp.214–215)

6 Sitting Twist (see pp.222–223)

5 midweek
boost

Here is a strong sequence to pick you up when your energy starts to flag in the middle of the week. Start with Sectional Breathing (see p.149) and some breathe-and-stretch exercises of your choice (see p.150). Then do the postures shown here. Try using Audible Breath (see p.224) throughout the program.

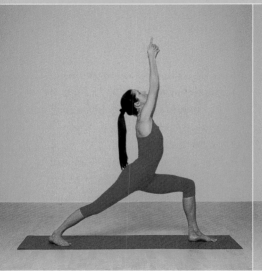

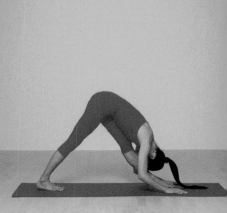

1 Warrior (see pp.164–165)

2 Runner's Stretch (see pp.186–187)

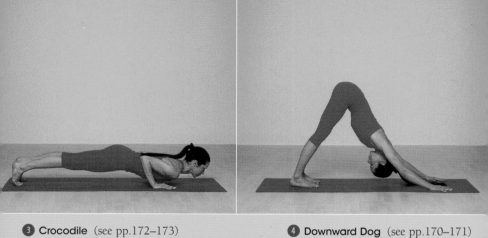

③ **Crocodile** (see pp.172–173)

④ **Downward Dog** (see pp.170–171)

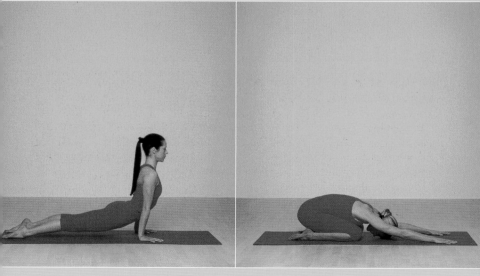

⑤ **Upward Dog** (see pp.174–175)

⑥ **Hare** (see pp.200–201)

6 weekend
energizer

Here is an invigorating routine that will set you up for the whole weekend. Integrate the postures with breathe-and-stretch exercises (see p.150), Sun Salute (see p.176), and the Kneeling Stretch sequence (see p.218). Add some breathing practices (see p.224) and the relaxation practice (see p.232) for a longer session.

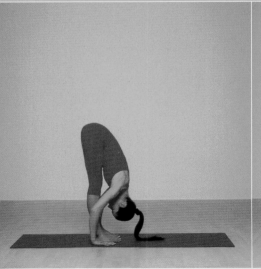

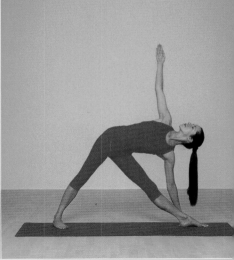

1 **Forward Bend** (see pp.162–163)

2 **Triangle** (see pp.182–183)

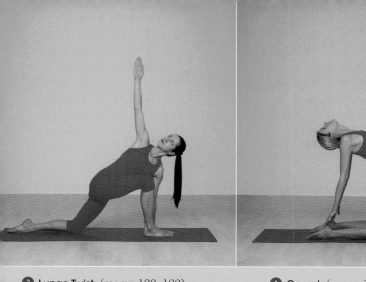

3 Lunge Twist (see pp.188–189)

4 Camel (see pp.202–203)

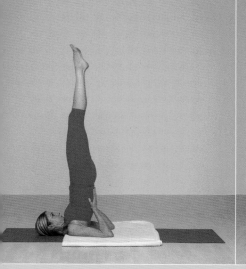

5 Full Shoulder Stand (see pp.208–209)

6 Sitting Forward Stretch (see pp.214–215)

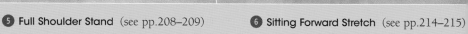

7 long journey reviver

To reduce the stress of long journeys, take frequent breaks during trips to breathe and stretch or to center yourself. At the end of a long journey, the Side-Bending sequence (see p.192), the Kneeling Stretch sequence (see p.218) and the following postures will all help you to unwind. End the program with the relaxation practice (see p.232).

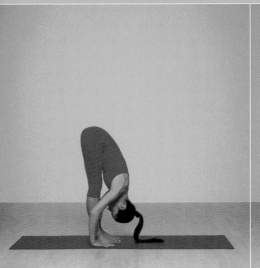

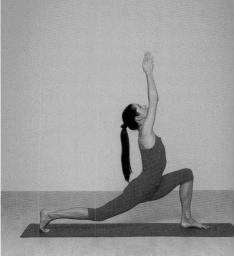

1 Forward Bend (see pp.162–163)

2 Lunge Warrior (see pp.166–169)

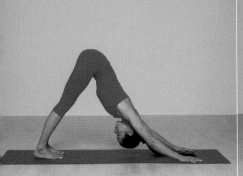

3 Downward Dog (see pp.170–171)

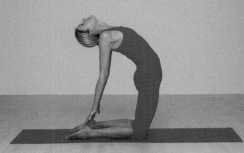

4 Camel (see pp.202–203)

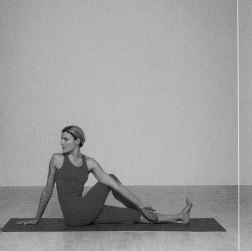

5 Sitting Twist (see pp.222–223)

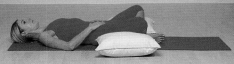

6 Supine Butterfly (see pp.216–217)

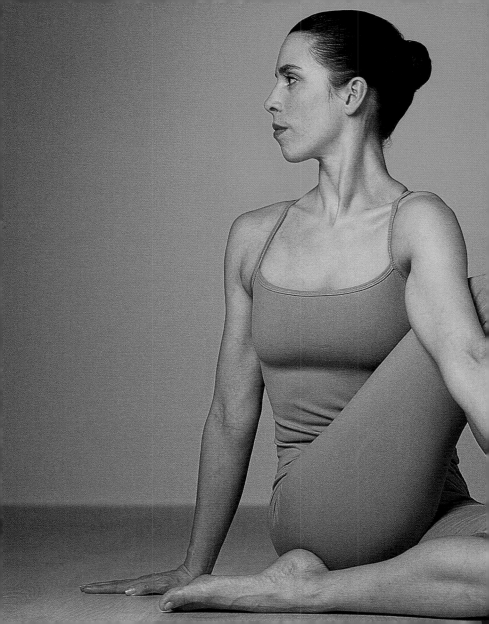

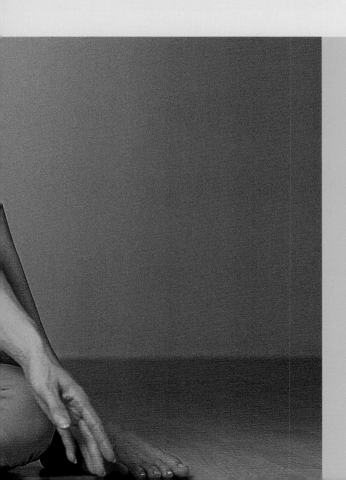

young

staying
young

The holistic practices of yoga work on the physical, mental, emotional, and spiritual planes, helping you live more positively and actively, and enabling you feel and look younger for longer.

The continuing improvements that are being made in medical science, health care, and living conditions mean that people today are living longer than at any time in the past. A man born in the US at the start of the 21st century has a life expectancy of about 75 years, while a woman can expect to live to about 80 – this is nearly twice as long as someone born in the mid-19th century. Because we now live longer, we have become more concerned about growing old. There is a desire to hold back the passage of time, to find ways of staying young so that we can enjoy our longer lives to the full.

Yoga can help us achieve this goal through its holistic approach to healthy living. Its combination of physical postures, breathing practices, relaxation, meditation, and lifestyle guidance can help you to stay physically fit, mentally alert, as well

HEALTH CONCERNS

If a health practitioner has advised you not to over-exert yourself physically, or if you have any other health concerns, seek advice from a qualified yoga therapist or teacher (see p.495) before using this book. Page 9 provides basic advice for some common medical conditions and, where appropriate, "Take Care" advice and "Alternatives" are given for individual practices. If you are pregnant, or have recently given birth, ask a suitably qualified yoga teacher which practices would be appropriate for you.

Practicing yoga regularly will nourish your mind, body, and spirit, helping to keep you fit and healthy, and making you feel and look younger than your years.

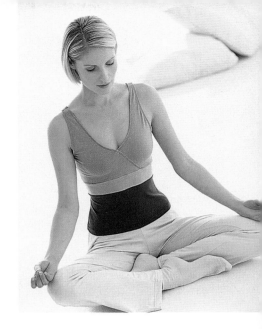

as help you to live more positively and more mindfully. By practicing yoga, you will be able to retain your vitality as you get older, and stay young at heart.

Unlike some forms of exercise, yoga is suitable for everyone. Whatever your age or level of fitness, yoga is a very safe form of exercise, provided you work within your limits. However, please read through the text below left, entitled "Health Concerns," before you begin your practice, because some yoga practices can be physically demanding.

What is aging?

Aging is a natural process, but there are different ways of looking at it. First, there is the passage of time itself: chronological aging. Then there are the physical changes that take place: biological aging. Finally, there is the matter of how we see ourselves: psychological aging.

Chronological age is often a poor guide to how old a person looks or feels. Everyone knows people who seem incredibly young for their age and others who almost seem to have been born old.

Biological aging follows a fairly predictable course. Our bodies tend, naturally, to be in prime condition when we are in our 20s. From then on, there is a slow, initially imperceptible but nevertheless inevitable, process of decline from that peak. Some of the key physical changes are noted below:

HORMONES AND MENOPAUSE

Generally speaking, our hormonal systems show comparatively few major changes with age. The big exception is the sharp fall in estrogen levels in the female body at the menopause, which typically occurs between 45 and 55.

The majority of physical side-effects experienced in the run up to menopause, such as hot flashes, night sweats, headaches, joint and muscle pains, and fatigue, are transitory (although they may not seem so at the time!), and very few women experience all of them. However, there are two important long-term side-effects. The first is that falling estrogen levels have been linked to osteoporosis; in extreme cases this can cause spinal curvature, the collapse of spinal vertebrae, and an increased risk of fractures. The second important side-effect is the loss of the relative protection from heart disease and strokes that women enjoy while their ovaries are still producing estrogen.

There is a great deal a woman can do for herself to help minimize the side-effects of menopause. She can eat a balanced diet and have a healthy, moderately active lifestyle that incorporates yoga practice.

• From about the age of 30, bones start to become thinner, and there is a gradual loss of density and strength as the body's ability to absorb calcium declines.

• As early as 20, joint flexibility starts to decline as ligaments become less elastic, and for many, daily wear and tear on joint surfaces leads to arthritic changes later in life, which further inhibit joint mobility.

• In our 30s, muscle size, strength, and flexibility start to decline. Tolerance for exercise diminishes, and recovery from injuries takes longer and is less complete.

• Changes to heart muscle and blood vessels make the cardiovascular system progressively less efficient in responding to the demands of exercise. Cardiovascular disease rates rise sharply after the age of 50.

• Loss of lung tissue elasticity and lung damage, caused by, for example, pollutants, reduce respiratory capacity and exercise performance. Ribcage rigidity and poor breathing habits often compound these changes. Chronic bronchitis and other chronic obstructive airway diseases affect about 17 percent of men and 8 percent of women in the 40–65 age group.

• All our senses are affected with age; we become more far-sighted from about 40 on, less able to hear high-frequency sounds, and our sense of balance becomes less sure.

• By the age of 65 we have lost about 10 percent of the brain cells we had as a young adult. Short-term memory tends to suffer first; for example being unable to repeat telephone numbers and recall events that happened only recently. Our reflexes also become slower.

• The immune system gradually becomes less efficient at combating disease, and we become more susceptible to viruses and bacterial infections. Rates for many types of cancer start to rise after the age of 50.

Why do we age?

Biological aging occurs primarily because, as the years pass, our body's cells become less and less efficient. The genetic material within each cell suffers increasing damage, which the cell finds harder and harder to repair.

The activity of special molecules, known as free radicals, is believed to be particularly important in causing cell damage. Many free radicals are produced as a result of natural chemical processes in the body, but environmental pollution, smoking, and (possibly) additives in foodstuffs are also important influences. The body has excellent defenses against free radicals, but as you grow older, they become less effective.

Although biological aging is inevitable, the pace of changes varies enormously between individuals. To some extent, it depends on your genes; some people have more robust defense and repair mechanisms than others. Genetic factors also play a part in many age-related conditions, such as high blood pressure, coronary heart disease, osteoarthritis, late-onset diabetes, and some cancers. But hereditary predisposition does not imply inevitability. Lifestyle factors, such as the extent to which you exercise, whether or not you smoke, the quality of your diet, staying mentally alert, and how you handle stress, have a very important role in determining the pace at which your body ages. The same is true of environmental factors. To give a very simple example, the rate at which your skin ages is greatly influenced by how much you are exposed to the sun and to environmental pollutants.

Your psychological age can be affected by your chronological age – but only if you let it – and by how

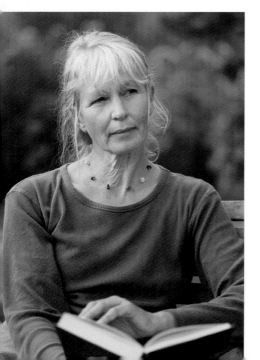

your body has fared with time. But your attitudes can also have a powerful influence on how you age physically. If you think of yourself as old simply because you have reached a certain age, you are more likely to age more rapidly physically as well as mentally. Attitude is all-important. A positive outlook on life, a cheerful disposition, feeling good about yourself, appreciating the world and other people, having goals, and having a flexible attitude can all help you to stay young at heart.

How can yoga help?

Yoga can make an important contribution to helping people stay feeling young and healthy.

Many studies in recent years have highlighted the benefits of moderate exercise: improved aerobic endurance, balance, and coordination; stronger muscles, increased flexibility, and better reaction time; and an overall

Yoga can bring a sense of inner calm, which will help you to face life's many challenges positively, and to get more out of life as the years pass.

feeling of physical and mental well-being. Medical advice is that you should exercise moderately for a minimum of 30 minutes a day. Three sets of 10 minutes is just as good as 30 minutes, and for those who lead sedentary lives, this approach may be better when first practicing yoga.

Yoga's combination of physical postures and breathing and relaxation practices helps to nourish all the systems in our body. Its mix of moving and held postures is particularly suited to relieving muscular tension and increasing flexibility, muscular strength, and joint mobility. Weight-bearing poses can help to maintain strong bones. Improved posture leads to a more positive and youthful self-image.

Yoga can be used to develop aerobic stamina through dynamic sequences, such as the Sun Salute (see p.324). It is also completely compatible with other activities that provide cardiovascular exercise, such as walking, dancing, and swimming. Yoga encourages you to respect your body by eating healthily and making sure you get enough rest.

Lifestyle changes

Yoga is not just a particular form of physical exercise. The fundamental aim is to enable you to find the calm, quiet core of your being – to "still the thought waves of the mind," as Patanjali, a great yoga master, put it so well more than 2,000 years ago. All yoga practices, and in particular breathing practices and meditation, can help you to let go of physical, mental, and emotional distractions.

Bringing yoga into your daily life encourages you to live in the present, to be with "what is" and, as a consequence, to be able to see more clearly and act mindfully, giving your full attention to whatever you are doing or to whoever you are with.

To do this, you need to be prepared to examine your habitual patterns of behavior. For example, how often do you label and categorize yourself and other people in agist terms and act according to preconceived stereotypes? How often do you give in to negative emotions, such as anger, fear, and envy? Do you have a tendency to cling to the past and what might have been for too long, or live hoping (or fearing) about what the future might bring?

Yoga encourages you to let go of these energy-sapping attitudes and emotions and replace them with more positive attitudes. For example, treating other people with respect and compassion; being honest with yourself; shunning feelings of jealousy and being content with the simple things in life, rather than always seeking to possess more.

Women and yoga

Developing a positive approach to life, as advocated by yoga, keeping active through physical yoga practices, and finding your calm center through relaxation and meditation can be particularly helpful for women in the run up to and during menopause.

For many women, menopause can be a potentially dispiriting time. Aside from the physical side-effects

MAXIMS FOR LIVING

A positive relationship with the world and with yourself was of fundamental importance to Patanjali. Try to live by his maxims (interpreted below). They will help you to live more positively, allowing life energy to flow more freely through you.

In your relationship with the world around you, you should:
• Avoid causing harm; endeavor to be compassionate.
• Be honest in all your thoughts, words, and actions.
• Never steal from others. This applies not only to possessions but also to wasting other people's time, energy, and goodwill.
• Be faithful and selfless in all your personal relationships.
• Avoid acquiring or holding on to material things (or people) for the sake of it, or for selfish reasons.

In relation to yourself, you should work to:
• Develop purity in mind, body, and spirit – inner and outer cleanliness.
• Pursue simplicity in life, and try to make the most of whatever life brings.
• Develop physical and mental resolve (through yoga practices) to withstand difficulties and disappointments in life.
• Learn to identify with your inner self rather than with your habitual ways of acting and seeing situations.
• Accept that there is more to life than the material world, and be respectful of the intelligence underpinning life.

(see p.254), menopause can be emotionally challenging. If it is seen as an unambiguous signal of a loss of role in life – that is, the loss of ability to conceive – and of embarking on the downward path of aging, then the experience and long-term effects are likely to be negative. If, on the other hand, women refuse to accept this stereotype imposed by society, and menopause is viewed as simply another stage in a life that has many years yet to run, it can provide opportunities for increased independence and new directions. The experience is then more likely to be positive, and not a milestone in the aging process.

The right attitude

Having the willpower to exercise regularly is not easy for many people, and changing attitudes, as advocated by yoga, can be even more challenging. But it is possible to make these changes, and the benefits of doing so in terms of increased vitality, peace of mind, and maintaining a youthful outlook on life, make it well worth the effort.

HOW TO USE THIS SECTION

Young is divided into three sub-sections. **Foundations** provides guidance on doing yoga and some basic breathing and preliminary stretches. Familiarize yourself with these first before moving on to **Building Blocks**. This contains a selection of postures and breathing practices, as well as a simple meditation and relaxation technique. Work through these postures gradually, selecting one or two to work on at a time, rather than trying to do them all in at once. Look at the photographs first to get a feel for the overall shape of the posture. Then follow the accompanying step-by-step instructions carefully. If you find a posture difficult to do, work on the preliminary steps first or try the alternative, if one is given.

Programs combines selected postures and other practices in a series of short yoga programs designed for particular situations and needs. Make sure you understand how to do the postures first before trying these programs.

Yoga is traditionally learned from a teacher, and you will benefit from going to a class, if you are not already doing so. Organizations that can help you find a qualified teacher are listed on page 495.

the basics

At the beginning of every posture, and linking some of them, is a basic standing, sitting, or lying position. Some examples of each, together with the use of some props, are shown here. If your body is not very flexible, or if you have problems with your balance, it can be very helpful to use a prop, such as a block, belt, or pillow, to make sure you do not strain your body.

Good posture

The basic standing position can be regarded as a posture in itself, encouraging stability and awareness. Learning how to stand well can also help with postural problems. Sitting comfortably, with your spine and head erect, is essential when doing breathing practices and meditation, enabling you to remain focused throughout. Being comfortable when lying down is crucial for relaxation.

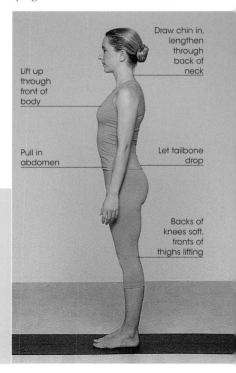

Draw chin in, lengthen through back of neck

Lift up through front of body

Pull in abdomen

Let tailbone drop

Backs of knees soft, fronts of thighs lifting

STANDING

Stand up straight with your feet parallel, hip-width apart, and your ears, tops of shoulders, hips, and ankles in line. Press your feet to the ground to lift upwards through the body. Broaden across the top of the chest. Feel balanced in all directions, with your head held as if it is suspended by a thread from the ceiling. Look ahead, relax, and breathe easily.

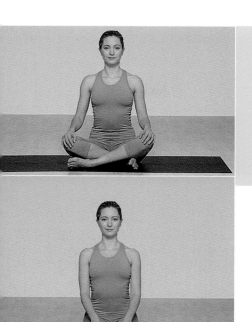

EASY SITTING

This basic posture is good for breathing practices. Cross your shins with each foot under the opposite knee. Position yourself on the front edge of your sitting bones, with the spine long and the head erect. Allow the hips to relax. If your knees are higher than your hips, sit on a block or another support.

KNEELING

If you find basic cross-legged sitting uncomfortable, sit on your heels with the tops of your thighs facing the ceiling. If you are going to be kneeling for a long time, place your knees and feet hip-width apart and sit on blocks, a folded blanket, or a bolster. Keep your spine long and head erect. Rest your hands on your thighs or in your lap.

LYING ON BACK

This posture is commonly used for relaxation. Lie on your back with your feet about hip-width apart, feet relaxing out, your arms slightly away from the sides of your body with the palms facing up, and the center of the back of your head resting on the floor.

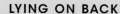

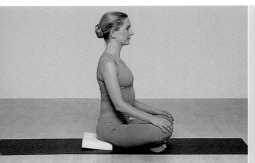

FOAM BLOCK

If your hips are stiff or your back tends to collapse when you are sitting, a foam block may help, as in Sitting Stretch (see p.340). If your neck is uncomfortable when you are lying on your back, you may find it useful to have a block as a support under your head.

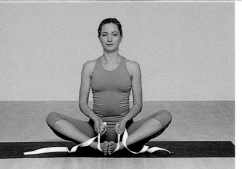

BELT

One of the most common uses for a belt is as an extension of the arms to help you avoid straining your back. In preliminary stretch, Hip Opener 3 (see p.283), use a belt to help keep the spine long and the shoulders relaxed as you take your knees toward the floor.

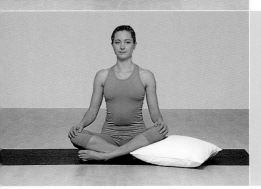

PILLOW

A pillow can be used instead of a block to sit on or to rest your head on. It can also be used as a support to help relieve muscular tension. In Sitting Stretch (see p.340) a pillow could be placed under the bent knees to help relieve tension in the inner thigh muscles.

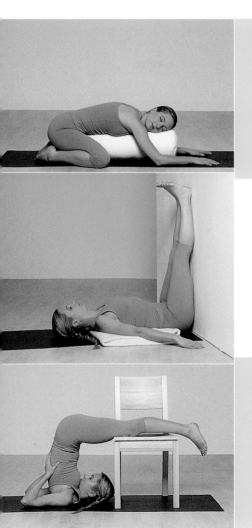

BOLSTER

A bolster can support you in various ways. For example, resting the upper body on a bolster in this wide-legged version of Child (see p.339) is very relaxing. Lying on your back with a bolster under the knees can be helpful if you have back problems.

BLANKET

A blanket can be used to keep warm in meditation and relaxation, and as a support, for example in the preparatory stage for Shoulder Stand Against a Wall, as shown here. A folded blanket, 3 ft (1 m) square, is positioned under the shoulders, so that in the final pose (see p.331) the shoulders are at the edge of the blanket but the neck is off it.

CHAIR

Apart from being used to sit on, a chair can be used to modify postures to provide support for different parts of the body. For example, in Plow (see p.336), you can use a chair if you lack the flexibility to take your feet to the floor. A chair can also be used for support if your balance is poor (see Tree on p.303).

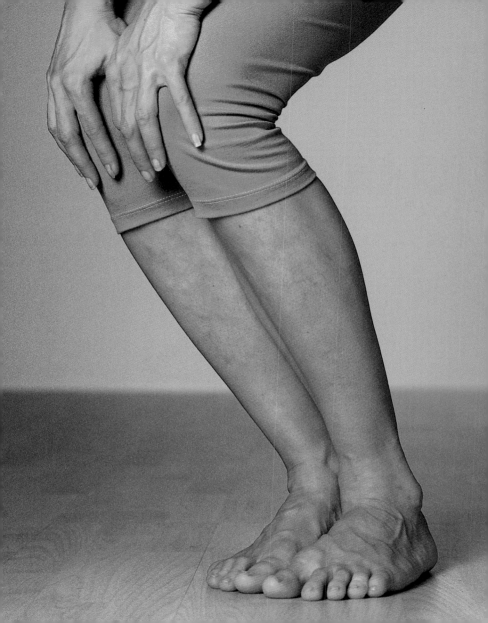

foundations

This section shows you basic standing, sitting, and lying postures. It provides breathe-and-stretch exercises to loosen your body and help you coordinate breath with movement. Breathing and centering practices are also given, bringing awareness to your yoga practice.

centering

When you practice yoga, your attention needs to be on the present moment. Centering is a simple technique to help you let go of distracting thoughts and emotions and bodily tensions.

You can center yourself by standing, sitting, or lying down quietly for a few minutes in a comfortable position. Simply observe your breath, letting it settle into a quiet, natural rhythm. As you do so, the activity in the mind will lessen. However, if your body is stiff and your muscles tense, you might find it helpful to do the supine centering relaxation practice detailed below before undertaking any postures.

becoming centered

1 Lie on the floor with your knees bent, feet hip-width apart. Place your arms away from the sides of the body, the backs of the hands on the floor, and the fingers gently curling inward. Position the center of the back of the head on the floor, and relax the neck. If your neck feels strained, try placing a small support (for example, a block, or thin pillow) under your head.

2 Allow your lower back to sink toward the floor. Slide your feet along the floor to stretch the legs out. Let the legs relax and the feet fall out. (If you feel discomfort in your back, keep your knees bent.) Close your eyes. Be aware of how balanced your body feels. Are the different parts of the body sinking into the floor equally or are there tensions or restrictions in some areas?

3 Slowly take your attention to each part of your body and let it relax. Start with the feet and work slowly up through the lower legs, upper legs, hips, buttocks, hands, lower arms, upper arms, chest, back, shoulders, neck, and face. Feel each part of the body releasing down to the floor in turn. Then become aware of your breath. Make sure you are breathing through your nostrils. Do not try to control the breath or change it in any way; simply observe its movement in and out of the body. Let the breath settle into a slow, deep, natural rhythm. Each time you breathe out, be aware of letting go. Feel the body "sinking" into the floor, but at the same time feel that it is supported by the floor.

4 Bring your attention to your out-breath. Allow it to become a little longer than your in-breath. Now count 10 out-breaths. The breath should remain calm and unhurried as you count. When you reach zero, gently turn the head from side to side three times. Then, on an in-breath, stretch your arms up and over your shoulders to the floor behind you. Stretch through to the fingertips, and press your lower back to the floor and your heels gently toward the wall in front of you. Relax into the stretch for a few breaths. Then, on an out-breath, bring your arms back down to your sides. Let go completely. Slowly turn onto one side of your body, pause for a few breaths, then slowly sit or stand up.

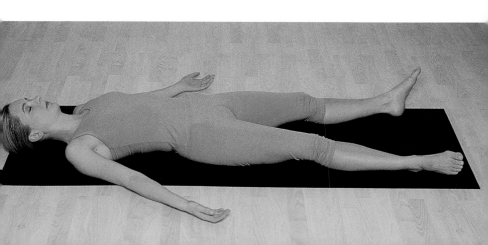

basic breathing

Breathing well is of fundamental importance to our physical, mental, and emotional health. In yoga, the breath is how vital energy – "the breath behind the breath" – enters the body.

Breathing provides oxygen for the metabolic processes from which we derive the energy to move, think, and feel. It also carries away carbon dioxide, the main waste product of metabolism. Physical tension in the respiratory muscles between and around the ribs can cause tightness in the chest, and even chest pain. Relaxed breathing techniques will release tension from the whole of the upper body, including the neck and shoulders. This will improve your ability to adjust your breathing to meet changing requirements.

The breath also provides a powerful link between mind and body. By controlling your breathing patterns – for example, the rhythm and depth of breathing, the length of the out-breath, and the balance between the right and left nostrils – you can influence your physical, mental, and emotional states.

Good breathing habits

Yoga encourages breathing through the nose, full use of the diaphragm, a slow, smooth breathing pattern, and coordination of movement and breath. Opening movements, such as back bends, are practised on an in-breath, and closing movements, such as forward bends, on an out-breath.

The breathing practice on the next page will help develop awareness of the action of respiratory muscles and encourage good breathing habits. It can be done standing or sitting, as well as lying down.

sectional breathing

Sectional breathing helps unlock energy blocks associated with poor breathing habits. After completing

Step 3, combine all three steps to produce full, continuous in-breaths and out-breaths.

1 Lie down with your knees bent, your palms resting on the abdomen. Breathe into your hands, feeling the abdomen swell out and the fingers move apart as you breathe in. Then, feel the abdomen sink back as you exhale. Take six even breaths.

2 Bring your hands to your lower ribs, with your fingers to the front and thumbs on the back ribs. Feel the ribs expand into the hands on the in-breath and relax back inward as you exhale. Take six breaths like this.

3 Place your fingers on the collarbones, in front of your shoulders. Breathe in and feel the top of the chest expand and the fingers rise up toward the head. As you breathe out, feel the chest and fingers sink back down. Take six breaths like this.

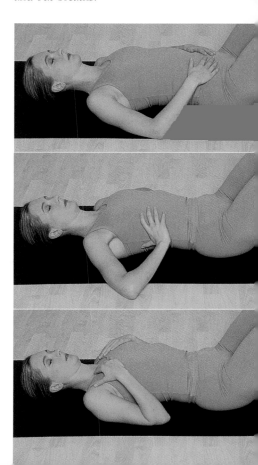

preliminary stretches

These gentle stretches will help ease stiff muscles and joints before you go on to more demanding postures. They will also help you become more aware of coordinating movement with breath.

knee circling

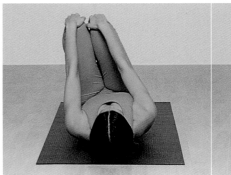
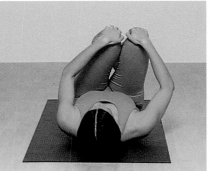

1 Lie on your back with your knees bent, legs together. Lift your feet off the floor and place your hands on your knees. Breathing easily, circle the knees clockwise. Keep the circles small to begin with and the movement slow and smooth.

2 Keeping the breath and upper body relaxed, slowly make the circles larger as the back muscles release. After a while, change direction. Start with large circles and gradually make them smaller. Release the feet back to the floor. Relax.

head to knee

1 Lie on your back. Bring your right knee over the chest and clasp your hands just below the knee. Keeping the shoulders relaxed, ease the knee toward the chest on the out-breath.

2 Push the left heel away. On an out-breath, draw the abdomen in, tuck in the chin, and lift the head and shoulders off the floor. Breathe easily. After several breaths, lower the head to the floor and release the leg. Repeat with the left leg.

3 Bring both knees over the chest. If you have a back problem, do this one knee at a time, or stay with Step 1 or 2. Clasp the hands just below both knees, and keep the shoulders down away from the ears.

4 On an out-breath, draw the abdomen in and lift the head toward the knees. Breathe into the lower abdomen and exhale fully. Stay for several breaths, then lower your head slowly to the floor and release the knees. Relax.

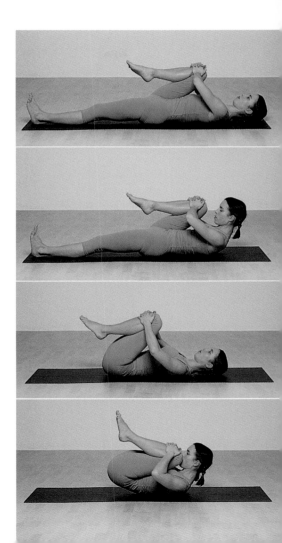

hamstring stretch

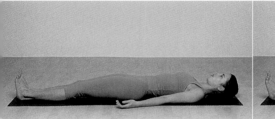

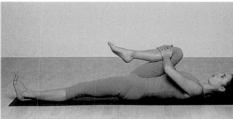

1 Lie on the floor with the legs stretched out in front. Lengthen the legs away from the hips and push through the heels.

2 Bring the right knee over the chest and clasp the shin with both hands. Slowly ease the knee closer to the chest on the out-breath. Push the left heel away.

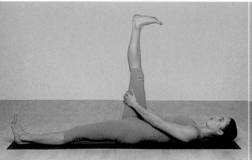

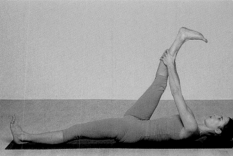

3 Slide your hands to the back of the thigh. Extend the leg up, pressing the heel away from you. Breathe easily as you lengthen through the back of the leg. If your knee remains bent, try the alternative (see opposite).

4 If Step 3 is easy, slide the hands toward the foot. On an out-breath, ease the straight leg toward the chest. Hold the position, breathing easily. Bend the knee again and lower your leg to the floor. Repeat on the left.

alternative hamstring stretch

1 If your hamstrings are tight, bring the right knee over the chest and loop a belt around the sole of your foot, holding opposite ends of the belt on each side of the leg.

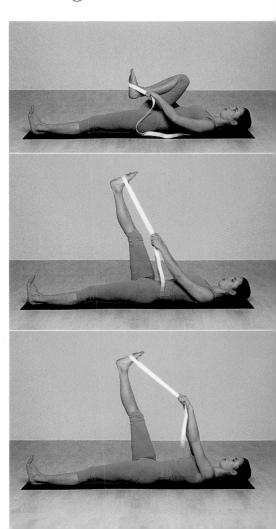

2 Extend the leg toward the ceiling. If your knee remains bent, allow the leg to come away from the upper body until it is straight. Push the heel away from you to lengthen through the back of the leg and feel the slight resistance against the belt.

3 Breathe easily, keeping the shoulders relaxed. On an out-breath, lift the arms and draw the belt toward your head, increasing the stretch through the back of the leg. Hold for several breaths. Bend the knee again to come out of the pose. Repeat on the left.

arm slide

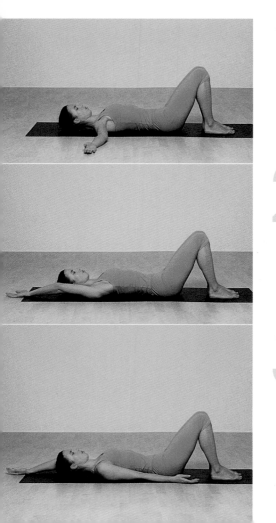

1 Lie with your knees bent. Take your arms out to the side at shoulder level, palms facing up. Breathe easily, then breathe in deeply and exhale fully, drawing the abdomen back toward the spine. Keep the abdomen held in as you continue to breathe in and out.

2 On an in-breath, slide your right arm up toward your head and your left arm down beside your hip. Let the breath guide the movement, and try to keep the back of the hand and the forearm touching the floor all the way. Pause briefly.

3 As you breathe out, slide the arms in the opposite direction so the left arm is now beside the head and the right arm at your side. Again, pause briefly. Repeat up to 10 times, then reverse the sequence: breathe in as you take the left arm up beside the head and the right arm down to the side. To finish, relax the abdomen, stretch your legs out, bring both arms down, and breathe freely.

hip lift

1 Lie on your back with the knees bent, hip-width apart, and heels beneath the knees. Lengthen through the back of the neck and have the center of the back of your head on the floor. Place your arms by your sides, palms facing down. Draw the shoulders away from the ears. Take several deep breaths.

2 On an in-breath, press your feet into the floor and lift the hips off the floor, bringing your weight onto your shoulders but keeping the neck free. As you exhale, take your tailbone toward your knees. Lift again on the in-breath and extend on the out-breath. Then hold, breathing into the abdomen. Keep the legs strong.

3 Come down slowly on an out-breath or, to take the pose farther, interlock your fingers behind your back and stretch the backs of the hands towards your feet. Hold the hips higher than the chest, the knees parallel, and your heels beneath the knees. Breathe deeply. To come out, release the hands and, on an out-breath, lower the back to the floor, one vertebra at a time. Relax for a few breaths.

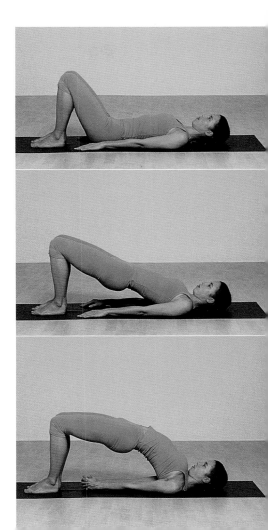

lying twist

1 Lie on your back with your knees bent, legs and feet together, and arms out to the side at shoulder level, with the palms facing up. If there is any discomfort in your neck, place a block or thin pillow under your head. Breathe easily.

2 As you exhale, let your knees drop to the right, keeping the knees and inner ankles together, and the outside of your right foot on the floor. At the same time, turn your head to the left and press the left shoulder into the floor. Do not worry if your knees do not reach the floor. Never try to force them down.

3 On an inhalation, bring the knees and head slowly back to face the ceiling. On the out-breath take the knees to the left and the head to the right. In the twist, relax and focus on the movement of the breath in your abdomen and ribcage.

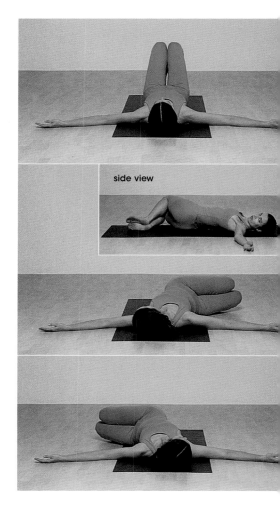

side view

joint mobilization

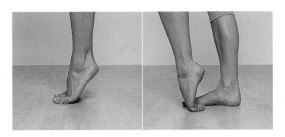

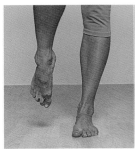

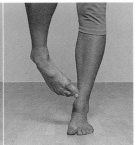

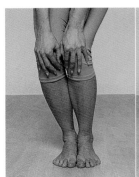

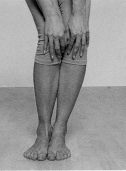

TOES

Rise up and down on your toes a few times. Then roll onto the front of one foot to gently press the toes into the floor. Hold for a few breaths, then repeat with the other foot.

ANKLES

Lift one foot off the floor and rotate it gently in both directions, describing large circles with the big toe. Repeat with the other foot. Keep the supporting leg as still as possible.

KNEES

Stand with the feet and legs together. Bend the knees and hold onto the kneecaps with your fingers pointing down. Rotate your knees 10 to 20 times clockwise and then 10 to 20 times counterclockwise.

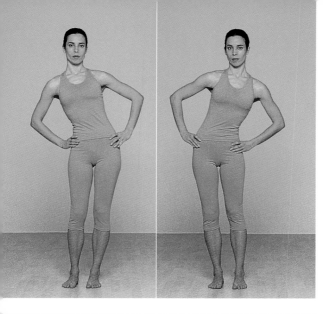

HIPS

With the feet about hip-width apart and your hands on your hips, circle the hips clockwise and then counterclockwise 10 to 20 times each way. Try to keep your knees still.

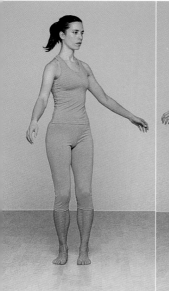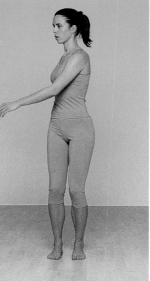

TORSO

Stand with your feet hip-width or more apart. Swing the arms freely from side to side, allowing the upper body to turn with the arms. Start with small, slow movements and then allow them to become larger and faster as the momentum builds. Build up cautiously if you have back problems.

WRISTS

Make fists with both hands, tucking the thumbs in. Holding the arms out in front of you and keeping them still, circle hands and wrists clockwise and counter-clockwise up to 10 times. Make the circles as smooth and as large as possible.

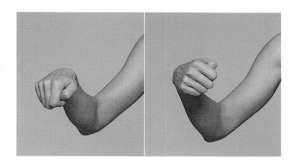

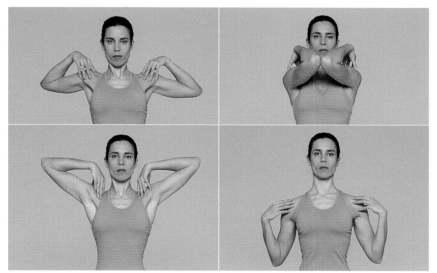

SHOULDERS

Standing, bring your fingertips onto your shoulders. As you breathe in, bring the elbows together in front of you and, keeping them together, lift them up. As you exhale, circle the elbows out, back, and down. On the in-breath, bring them forward and together again, and repeat Steps 2 to 4 five to 10 times.

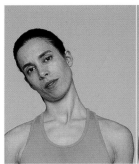
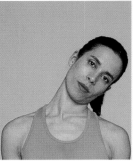

NECK

Stand or sit looking straight ahead, and draw your chin in slightly. On an out-breath, take your right ear slowly towards your right shoulder. Hold for three slow breaths. Feel the stretch. Come back up on the in-breath. Repeat on the left side.

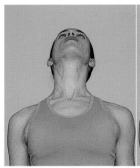
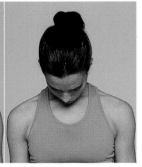

On an out-breath, take your chin toward the ceiling (but do not arch the neck back). Hold for three breaths. Come back on the in-breath. Then lower your chin toward your chest on the out-breath. Hold for three breaths. Come back up on the in-breath.

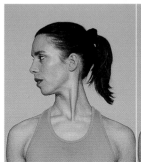
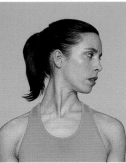

On the out-breath, turn your head slowly to the right, keeping your gaze at the same level throughout. Stay for three breaths. Come back to center on the in-breath and repeat on the left. Come back to center on an in-breath and breathe easily.

hip opener 1

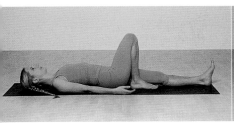

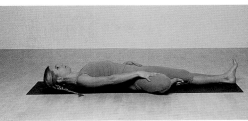

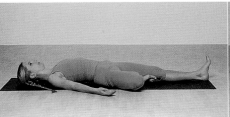

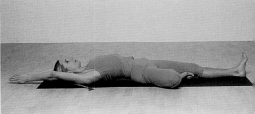

1 Lie on your back with your legs stretched out, arms by your sides. On an in-breath, draw your right leg up, sliding your foot along the floor until it is close to your buttock.

2 Bring the sole of the right foot against the left inner thigh as you lower the right knee toward the floor, pressing down gently with your right hand, if you need to. Use your left hand to help keep your left hip on the floor.

3 Keeping your left buttock on the floor, relax with your arms out to the side and breathe easily. To come out, raise the knee to vertical again on an in-breath and slide the foot along the floor to stretch the leg out. Repeat on the left side.

4 To extend the final position, bring the palms of your hands together on your chest and stretch the arms over your head. To come out, lower the arms to the side first, and then raise the knee and slide the leg away.

hip opener 2

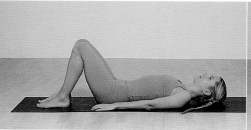

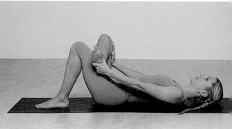

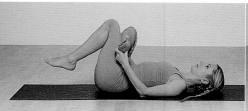

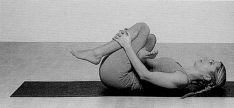

1 Lie on your back with the knees bent and hip-width apart. With your arms by your side, draw the shoulders down away from your ears. Make sure the center of the back of your head is on the floor.

2 Bring your right leg across your left thigh, so that the ankle joint clears the leg. Gently push the right knee away from you with your right hand. Hold your right foot steady with the left hand.

3 Bend the left leg toward you as you continue to push gently against the right knee with the right hand. Slowly swinging the left lower leg up and down will increase the stretch through the right buttock.

4 For a stronger stretch, slide the right hand between the legs and pull the left shin toward you with both hands (alternatively, use a belt). Stay relaxed and breathe easily. Release slowly and repeat on the left.

hip opener 3

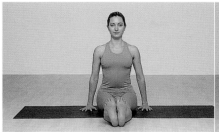

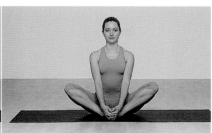

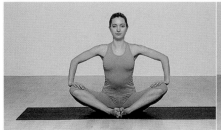

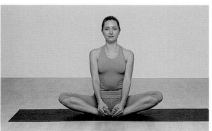

1 Sit with your legs stretched out. Press down onto the hands on each side of the hips to lengthen through the spine. If you cannot keep your legs straight, sit on a block.

2 Bring the soles of the feet together and pull them up as close to the groin as you can. Hold the feet with the hands. Breathe in and lengthen through the spine.

3 As you exhale, allow the knees to sink out to the side and down. If you are less flexible, try pressing down gently on the inner thighs with your hands. Breathe easily.

4 If you are more flexible, open the soles of the feet to the ceiling to bring the knees closer to the floor. To come out of the pose, raise the knees and stretch the legs out.

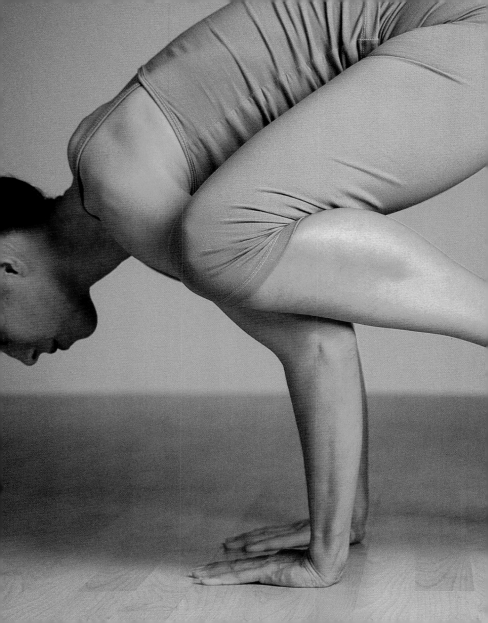

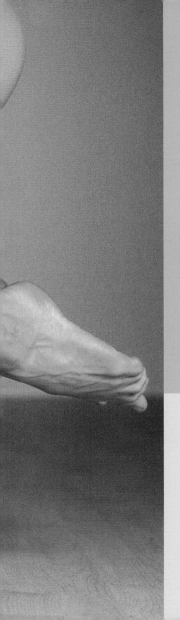

building blocks

These postures and practices will help release your inner strength and vitality. Work through them slowly, but not all at once! Become familiar with the steps and overall shapes, and then focus on becoming balanced and at ease while you practice them.

standing
side stretch

This quietly powerful sideways stretch for the upper body tones the postural and respiratory muscles, stimulating ribcage breathing and improving concentration. It is a good stretch to do at the office.

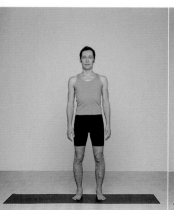 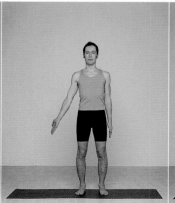 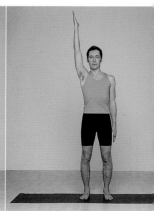

1 Stand up tall with your feet hip-width apart, arms by your sides, and shoulders relaxing down away from your ears. Look straight ahead and take several breaths.

2 On an in-breath, turn your right arm out, initiating the movement from the shoulder, so the whole arm turns, not just the hand.

3 Continuing to breathe in, extend the arm out to the side and up beside your head. Reach up for two or three breaths, keeping your weight balanced on both legs.

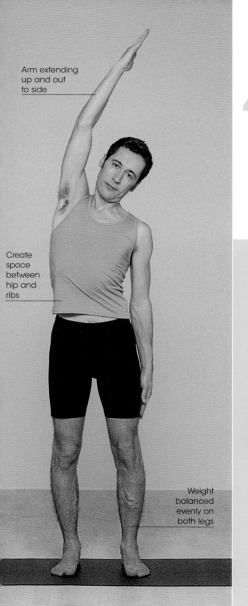

Arm extending up and out to side

Create space between hip and ribs

Weight balanced evenly on both legs

On an out-breath reach up and out to the left, keeping your head close to your arm. Press down through the sole of your right foot to stay balanced. Stay for several breaths, creating space between the top of the right hip and the ribs with each out-breath. Come back up on an in-breath and lower your arm on the out-breath. Repeat on the left side.

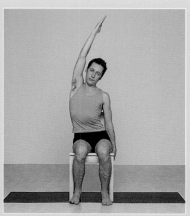

ALTERNATIVE

Sitting on a chair, circle your right arm up beside your head. Hold onto the seat with your left hand and lean to the right. At the same time, extend your right arm to the left. Stay for several breaths. Repeat on the left side.

lightning
bolt

This energizing posture helps tone the back and the abdominal muscles. It develops flexibility in the hips, knees, and ankles, and helps keep the legs young and strong.

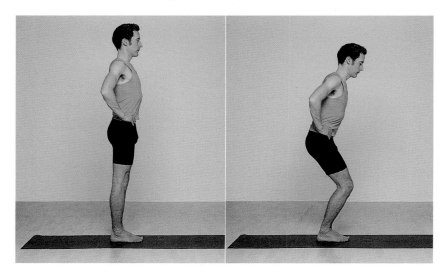

1 Stand with your feet together and your hands on your hips. Looking straight ahead, lift the top of the breastbone and breathe deeply.

2 On an out-breath, bend the knees and "sit back." Tuck the tailbone down, keeping your back long and your head in line with your body. Breathe deeply.

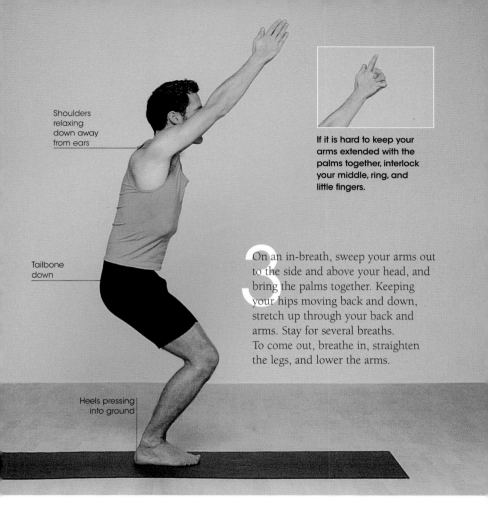

Shoulders
relaxing
down away
from ears

If it is hard to keep your
arms extended with the
palms together, interlock
your middle, ring, and
little fingers.

Tailbone
down

3 On an in-breath, sweep your arms out
to the side and above your head, and
bring the palms together. Keeping
your hips moving back and down,
stretch up through your back and
arms. Stay for several breaths.
To come out, breathe in, straighten
the legs, and lower the arms.

Heels pressing
into ground

TAKE CARE

• If you suffer from back pain, proceed cautiously.
• Keep your hands on your hips and hold the pose for
a short time only if you have HBP or a heart condition.

full
squat

Challenge the postural restrictions resulting from a life of sitting on chairs and promote flexibility in the hips, knees, and ankles. The squat also provides an invigorating stretch for the spine.

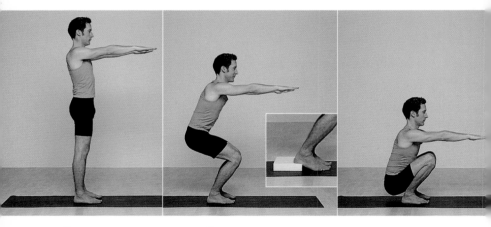

1 Stand with feet hip-width apart. Stretch the arms forward and breathe easily.

2 On an out-breath, bend your knees and start to "sit back." Keep your back long. If your heels lift off the floor, place a block under them.

3 Continue to "sit back," keeping your knees over your feet until you are squatting. Let your tailbone drop, keep lifting your breastbone, and breathe easily.

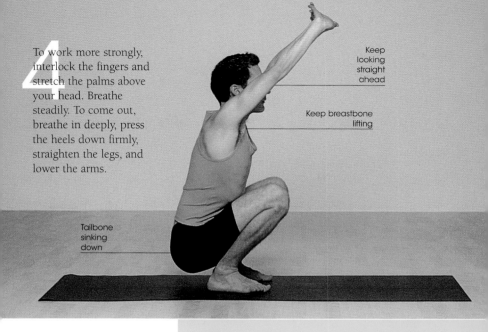

To work more strongly, interlock the fingers and stretch the palms above your head. Breathe steadily. To come out, breathe in deeply, press the heels down firmly, straighten the legs, and lower the arms.

Keep looking straight ahead

Keep breastbone lifting

Tailbone sinking down

TAKE CARE

• If you have back pain, proceed cautiously.
• Stop at Step 2 or do the alternative, using a chair if you have arthritic knees and hips, or are seriously overweight.
• Stop at Step 3 if you have HBP or suffer from a heart condition.

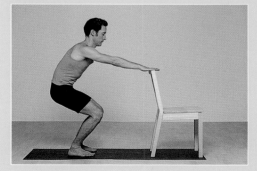

ALTERNATIVE

Rest your hands lightly on the back of a chair, table, or ledge to help you balance and stay in control as you "sit back" and as you come back up.

forward bend

Allow yourself to relax and let your spine release with this calming posture. Keep the feet rooted and the sitting bones lifting to help stretch tight hamstrings. Come out of the pose slowly.

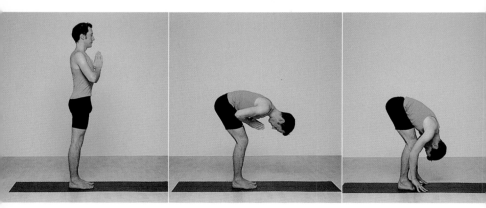

1 Stand with your feet hip-width apart. Bring the palms together in front of your chest. Draw the abdomen in and take a few breaths. Feel yourself broaden across the top of the chest and grow taller.

2 As you breathe out, bend your knees and fold forward from the hips. Keep your back as long as possible.

3 With your knees still bent, bring your fingers to the floor. Allow the spine to relax and lengthen as gravity pulls your head and upper body toward the floor.

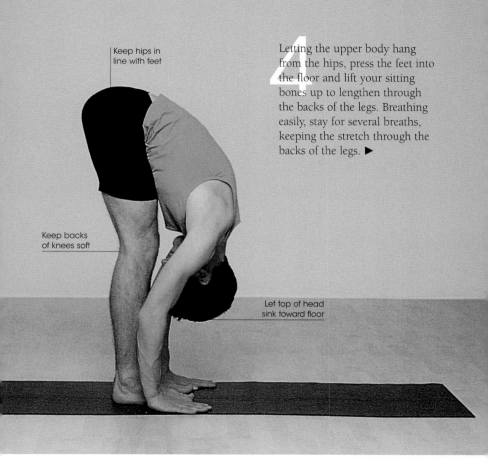

Keep hips in
line with feet

Letting the upper body hang
from the hips, press the feet into
the floor and lift your sitting
bones up to lengthen through
the backs of the legs. Breathing
easily, stay for several breaths,
keeping the stretch through the
backs of the legs. ▶

Keep backs
of knees soft

Let top of head
sink toward floor

TAKE CARE
• Proceed with caution and keep your knees bent
if you suffer from back pain.
• Do the Alternative pose (see p.294) if you have HBP,
heart disease, glaucoma, or a detached retina.

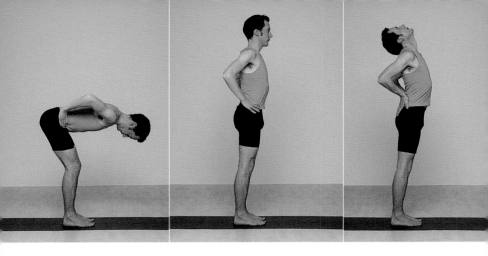

5 Bend both knees again and place your hands on your hips. On an in-breath, come up halfway, so that your upper body is parallel to the floor. Exhale and feel yourself lengthening through the spine.

6 On an in-breath, come all the way up, pivoting through the hip joints and keeping the back straight. As you breathe out, straighten your legs.

7 Slide your hands to the backs of your hips. As you breathe in, arch the back, opening the chest and lifting the chin (unless you have a neck problem). Stay for two more breaths, then straighten up again.

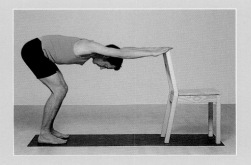

ALTERNATIVE

If you have HBP, heart disease, glaucoma, or a detached retina, do a Half Forward Bend using a chair. Pull the abdomen in gently, and keep the breastbone lifted and your head in line with the spine. Lengthen through the spine and the legs. Come back up on an in-breath, with the knees bent and a straight back.

forward bend &
back arch

Ideal for the office, this combined forward and back bend helps relieve tension in the back. It also encourages a full out-breath to leave you feeling revitalized and focused.

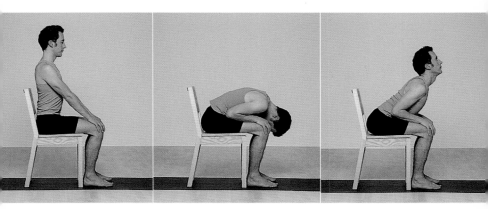

1 Sit up straight on a chair with the feet hip-width apart, the soles flat on the floor (place a block under your feet if you need to). Rest your hands on your kneecaps. Take several breaths.

2 Breathe in deeply. Then, as you exhale, lower your head to fold forward over the thighs, allowing your back to round.

3 As you breathe in, press your hands against your knees and lift your head, arching your back as you come back up. Repeat the sequence freely in a smooth flowing motion.

triangle

This posture builds strength and stability in the lower body and helps open the hips. Focus on your breath and feel the rejuvenating energy radiating out from your core through the arms, legs, and spine.

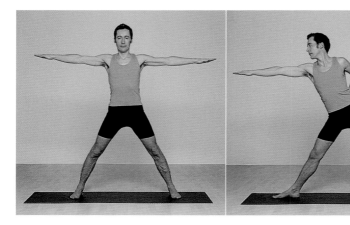

1 Start with your feet 3 ft (1 m) or more apart and your palms together, in front of your chest. On an in-breath, sweep your arms up and out to the sides at shoulder level. Relax the shoulders as you stretch through to the fingertips.

2 Turn your left heel out slightly and rotate the right leg from the hip until the toes point to the side. On an out-breath, reach out to the right and place the left palm on the back of the hips. Breathe in and push gently on the back to keep the left shoulder rotating back.

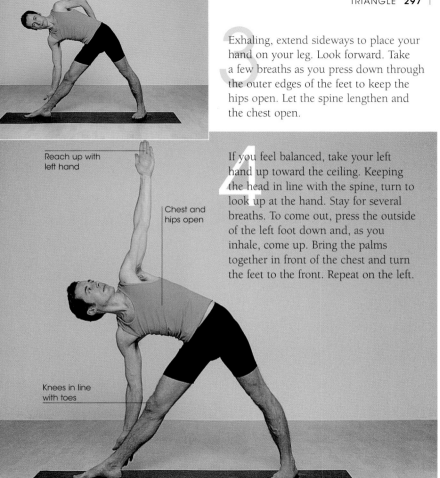

Exhaling, extend sideways to place your hand on your leg. Look forward. Take a few breaths as you press down through the outer edges of the feet to keep the hips open. Let the spine lengthen and the chest open.

If you feel balanced, take your left hand up toward the ceiling. Keeping the head in line with the spine, turn to look up at the hand. Stay for several breaths. To come out, press the outside of the left foot down and, as you inhale, come up. Bring the palms together in front of the chest and turn the feet to the front. Repeat on the left.

Reach up with left hand

Chest and hips open

Knees in line with toes

TAKE CARE
• HBP or heart disease: stop at Step 3. • Back problems: proceed with caution. • Neck problems: do not look up at hand.

side
warrior

This traditional posture promotes strength in the lower limbs and lower back, and flexibility in the hips. Use it when you need to feel strong and confident, balanced and focused.

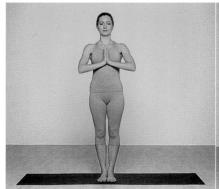 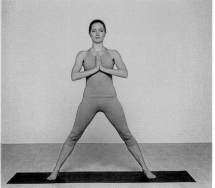

1 Stand with your feet together and bring your palms together, the thumbs touching the breastbone. With each in-breath, feel yourself lifting up through the body.

2 Step your feet 3 ft (1 m) or more apart. Keep the toes pointing forward. Press the outside edges of the feet down and feel the thigh bones rotate out. Let the tailbone drop. Breathe steadily.

TAKE CARE
• If you have HBP, or heart problems, stay in the posture for a short time only. • Proceed cautiously if you suffer from back pain.

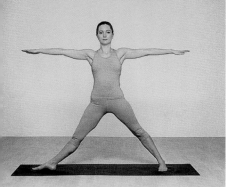

3 On an in-breath, sweep your hands up and out to the sides. Stretch through the arms and let the shoulders relax down. Pivot on the ball of the left foot to turn the heel out a little. Pivoting on the right heel, turn the right leg out, so the toes point to the side. Take several breaths and make sure you are balanced.

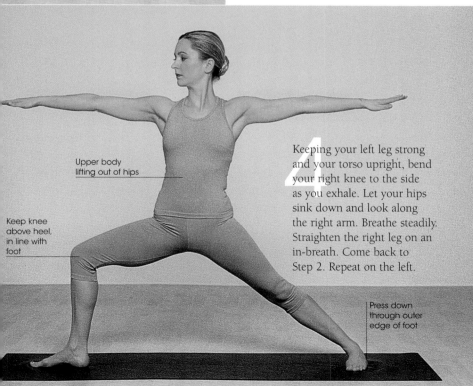

Upper body lifting out of hips

Keep knee above heel, in line with foot

4 Keeping your left leg strong and your torso upright, bend your right knee to the side as you exhale. Let your hips sink down and look along the right arm. Breathe steadily. Straighten the right leg on an in-breath. Come back to Step 2. Repeat on the left.

Press down through outer edge of foot

lunge warrior

In addition to providing a powerful stretch through the thigh and hip of the back leg, this pose extends the spine and opens the chest. Feel the vitality of the posture as you breathe deeply into the ribcage.

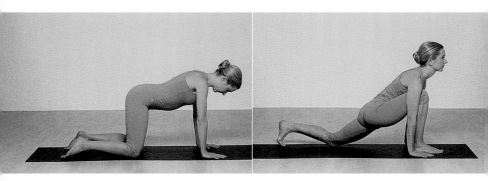

1 Begin on all fours, with the knees beneath the hips and the feet hip-width apart. Press the palms to the floor and stretch through the arms, bringing the shoulders away from the ears. Take several breaths.

2 On an in-breath, step the right foot forward between your hands (you may need to come on to your fingertips). Come onto the ball of your left foot. With your right knee directly above the heel, stretch through the upper body and look ahead. Breathe easily.

TAKE CARE
- If you have back problems, stop at Step 2 to begin with, if necessary.
- Do not hold the final position for long if you have HBP or heart problems.

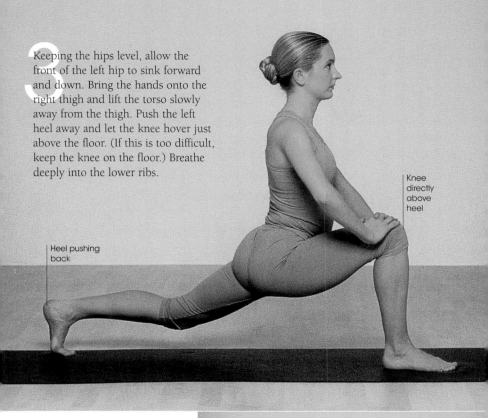

3 Keeping the hips level, allow the front of the left hip to sink forward and down. Bring the hands onto the right thigh and lift the torso slowly away from the thigh. Push the left heel away and let the knee hover just above the floor. (If this is too difficult, keep the knee on the floor.) Breathe deeply into the lower ribs.

Knee directly above heel

Heel pushing back

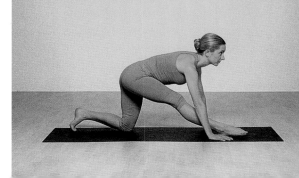

4 To come out, bring the left knee to the floor again and take the hips back to stretch through the back of the right leg. Slide your hands and right foot back to come into the all-fours position. Repeat on the left.

tree

Learning to maintain your balance in postures like Tree will help you keep a balance in life. Make sure you are firmly grounded by keeping the supporting leg strong and the foot firmly rooted.

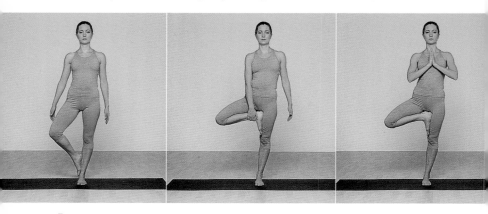

1 Stand with your feet together, arms by your side. Balancing on your left leg, bring the sole of your right foot onto the inside of the left calf. Press the left foot to the floor.

2 Slide the right foot up the inside of the left thigh. With the knee turned out, press your foot firmly against the leg. If you cannot keep the foot here, leave it as shown in Step 1.

3 Bring the palms together in front of the chest and keep the left leg strong. Look straight ahead and breathe evenly. Let the tailbone drop and lift the top of the breastbone.

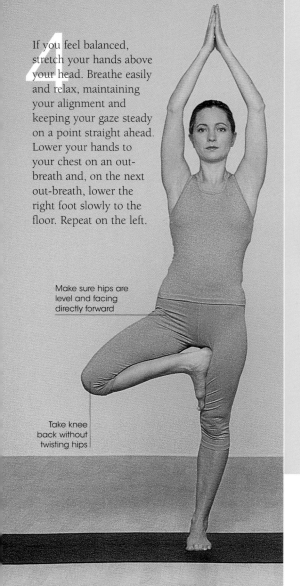

If you feel balanced, stretch your hands above your head. Breathe easily and relax, maintaining your alignment and keeping your gaze steady on a point straight ahead. Lower your hands to your chest on an out-breath and, on the next out-breath, lower the right foot slowly to the floor. Repeat on the left.

Make sure hips are level and facing directly forward

Take knee back without twisting hips

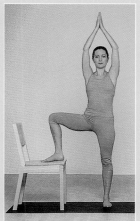

ALTERNATIVES

If your balance is poor, try facing a wall to aid concentration, or hold onto a chair to steady yourself. If you have arthritic hips or knees, or suffer from back problems, try the alternative pose shown above or leave the foot below the knee as in Step 1.

half
moon

A more advanced balancing posture that calls for strength in both legs and the back, and flexibility in the hips. Use a block and the wall to help you find your balance without fear of falling over.

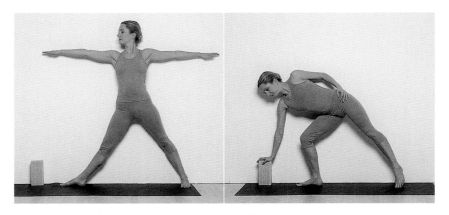

1 Stand close to a wall with your left foot turned slightly in and right foot parallel to the wall. Have a block a little away from your right foot.

2 On an out-breath, bend the right knee and, taking a small step in with the left foot, place your right hand on the block and rest your left hand on the front of your left hip.

TAKE CARE
- Avoid completely if you have back pain and the pose provokes symptoms.
- If you have neck problems, keep looking forward in the final pose.
- If you have HBP, or heart problems, keep your left hand on your hip.

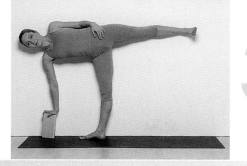

3 While straightening the right leg, raise the left leg parallel to the floor. Breathe in as you press down through the right foot, open the chest to the front, and rotate the left hip up and back. Relax the abdomen.

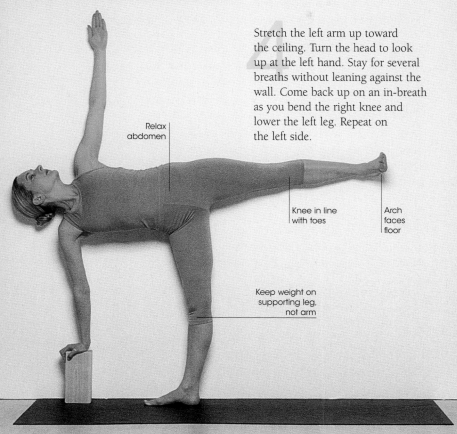

4 Stretch the left arm up toward the ceiling. Turn the head to look up at the left hand. Stay for several breaths without leaning against the wall. Come back up on an in-breath as you bend the right knee and lower the left leg. Repeat on the left side.

Relax abdomen

Knee in line with toes

Arch faces floor

Keep weight on supporting leg, not arm

crow

This weight-bearing posture for the wrists and arms requires you to stay focused, physically and mentally. Think of yourself as being as light as a bird, poised for flight, as you come into the balance.

1 Come into a squatting position, with the feet and knees shoulder-width apart, either by doing the Full Squat (see p.290) or by walking your hands back from an all-fours position. Bring the arms forward in front of the knees and place the hands on the floor with the fingers spread. Have the elbows bent and turned out.

TAKE CARE
• If you suffer back pain, avoid this pose if it provokes symptoms.
• If you have HBP, or heart problems, hold the final position only briefly.
• Stop at Step 2 if you have arthritis in wrists, glaucoma, or a detached retina.

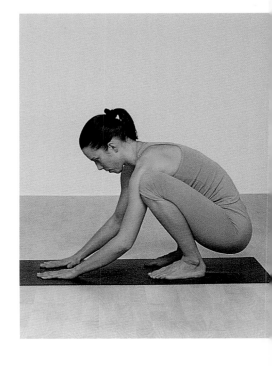

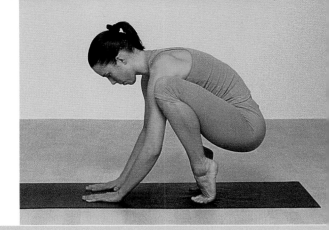

Focus your gaze on a point on the floor and breathe in deeply. Rising up on your toes, bring your weight forward over your hands as you exhale. Repeat several times to find your point of balance.

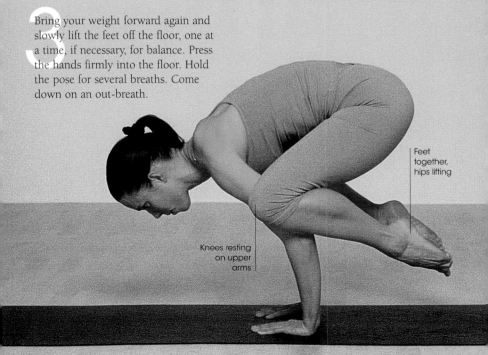

Bring your weight forward again and slowly lift the feet off the floor, one at a time, if necessary, for balance. Press the hands firmly into the floor. Hold the pose for several breaths. Come down on an out-breath.

Feet together, hips lifting

Knees resting on upper arms

cat

It is often said that you are as young as your spine. Keep your spine strong and flexible by arching your back like a cat. Focus on initiating the movement with your tailbone.

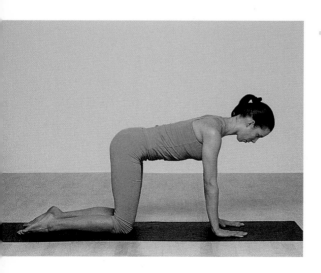

1 Start on all fours, with your knees under the hips. Keep the shoulders, elbows, and wrists in line, and the fingers spread. Bring the insides of the elbows to face each other, and lengthen through the arms as you bring the shoulders away from the ears. Keep the back in a relaxed straight line from the hips to the back of the head. Breathe easily.

TAKE CARE
• If your knees, hurt, try placing a folded towel under them.
• If you suffer from back pain, do the posture slowly to avoid provoking symptoms.

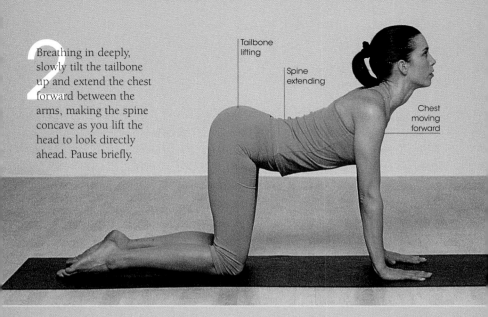

2 Breathing in deeply, slowly tilt the tailbone up and extend the chest forward between the arms, making the spine concave as you lift the head to look directly ahead. Pause briefly.

Tailbone lifting

Spine extending

Chest moving forward

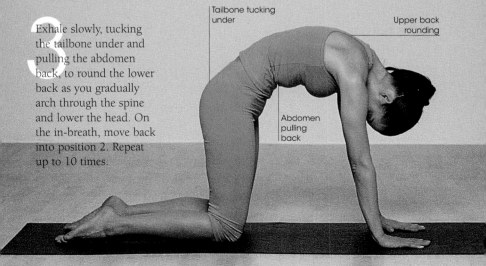

3 Exhale slowly, tucking the tailbone under and pulling the abdomen back, to round the lower back as you gradually arch through the spine and lower the head. On the in-breath, move back into position 2. Repeat up to 10 times.

Tailbone tucking under

Upper back rounding

Abdomen pulling back

cat
balance

This balance helps to develop stability in the hip and shoulder joints while stretching the body diagonally. Try to keep the back level, and be careful not to slump to one side.

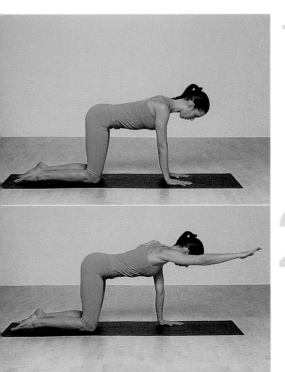

1 Start on all fours, with your knees under the hips. Keep the shoulders, elbows, and wrists in line, and the fingers spread. Bring the insides of the elbows to face each other, and lengthen through the arms as you bring the shoulders away from the ears. Keep the back in a relaxed straight line from the hips to the back of the head. Breathe easily.

2 Pull the abdomen back toward the spine and, as you breathe in, raise and stretch the right arm forward at shoulder height. Keep both shoulders level. Pause briefly, then lower as you breathe out. Repeat with the left arm. Do this several times on each side. Breathe easily.

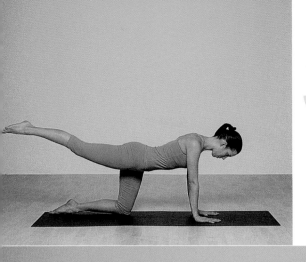

3 Pull the abdomen back and breathe in as you stretch the right leg back, pointing the toes away from you. Keep the hips level. Pause briefly, then lower the leg as you breathe out. Repeat with the left leg. Do this several times on each side. Breathe easily.

4 Draw the abdomen back and raise your right arm and left leg simultaneously as you breathe in. Pause briefly, then lower them as you breathe out. Repeat with the left arm and the right leg. Do several times on each side, then rest in Child pose (see p.338). Breathe easily.

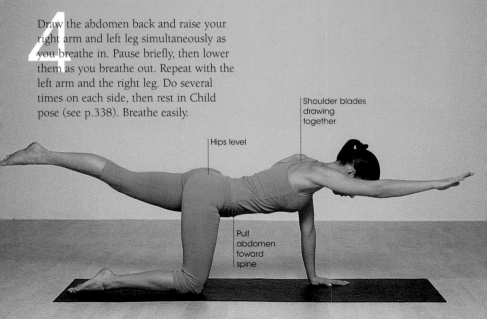

Hips level

Shoulder blades drawing together

Pull abdomen toward spine

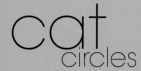

cat
circles

Combining balance with leg movements, this posture keeps the hip joints moving freely while strengthening the hip-stabilizing muscles. It also brings awareness and energy to the pelvic region.

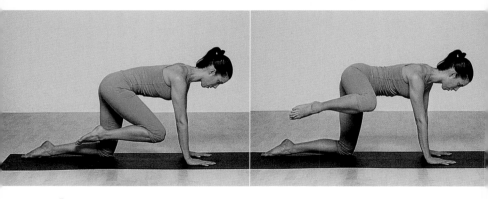

1 Start from the basic all-fours position (see Cat, p.308). Pull the abdomen in toward the spine, and as you breathe in, bring the knee forward toward the chest. Look down.

2 Continuing to breathe in and keeping the abdomen drawn in, start the circle by bringing the knee out to the side. Keep the hips as level as possible and the eyes looking down at the floor.

TAKE CARE
Make sure you keep the circles within the pain-free range of movement in the joint if you suffer from arthritis.

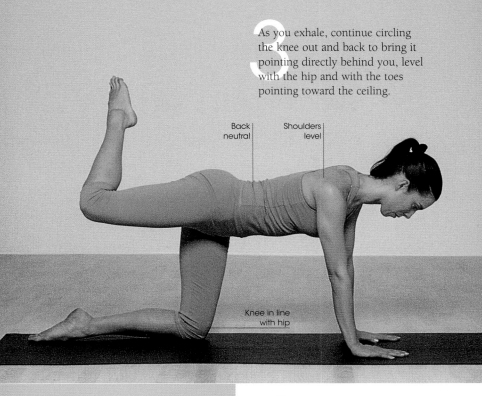

3 As you exhale, continue circling the knee out and back to bring it pointing directly behind you, level with the hip and with the toes pointing toward the ceiling.

Back neutral

Shoulders level

Knee in line with hip

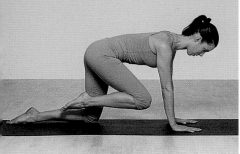

4 As you breathe in again, bring your knee forward to complete the circle. Repeat several times, keeping the circular movement flowing and even. Try to keep the shoulders and the left hip still. Repeat with the left leg.

downward
dog

This calming inversion, in which you stretch from the base of your fingers and the heels of your feet to your sitting bones, balances the upper and lower body, while strengthening the wrists, arms, and legs.

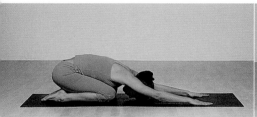

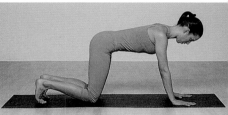

1 Sit on your heels, with your knees and feet hip-width apart. Slide your hands forward to come into the position shown. Spread the fingers.

2 Come up on all fours. Check that the hands are shoulder-width apart and ahead of the shoulders. Tuck your toes under. Take several breaths.

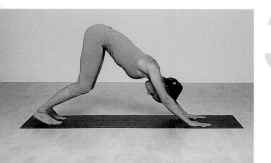

3 Take a deep breath in. Tilt your tailbone up, and as you exhale, press down with the base of the fingers and the balls of the feet to bring your knees off the floor, and lift your hips up and back, keeping your knees bent.

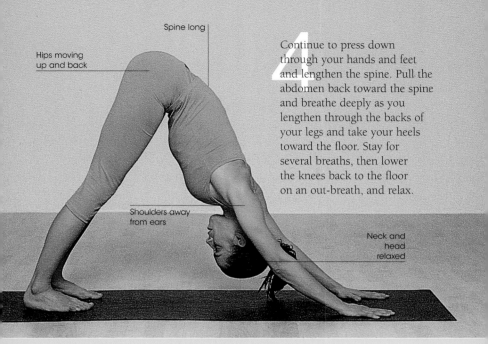

Hips moving
up and back

Spine long

4 Continue to press down
through your hands and feet
and lengthen the spine. Pull the
abdomen back toward the spine
and breathe deeply as you
lengthen through the backs of
your legs and take your heels
toward the floor. Stay for
several breaths, then lower
the knees back to the floor
on an out-breath, and relax.

Shoulders away
from ears

Neck and
head
relaxed

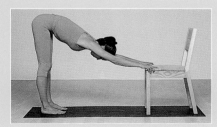

ALTERNATIVE

If you have HBP, heart problems,
glaucoma, or a detached retina, from
the basic standing position (see p.260),
hinge forward from the hips and place
your hands on the seat or back of a
chair. Lengthen through the backs of
the legs and stretch through the spine.

TAKE CARE

If you have back problems and/or tight hamstrings,
keep your knees bent in the final posture.

cobra

In this invigorating posture, you rise up like a cobra, extending the spine, strengthening the back muscles, and stimulating circulation to the spinal region. As the chest opens, feel the energy rising.

1 Lie on your front, forehead on the floor and feet hip-width apart. Place your hands under the shoulders and spread your fingers, the middle finger pointing forward. Keep the elbows close to the body and tuck your tailbone under.

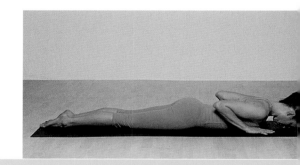

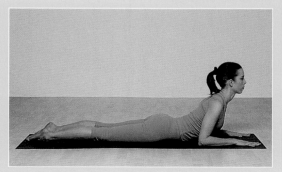

ALTERNATIVE

If you have HBP, heart disease, a hernia, or back or neck problems, start with your forearms on the floor, your hands beside your head. Press the elbows down as you lift the head and shoulders away from the floor on an in-breath. Lower on the out-breath.

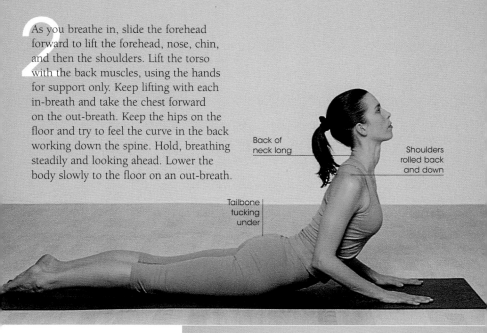

2 As you breathe in, slide the forehead forward to lift the forehead, nose, chin, and then the shoulders. Lift the torso with the back muscles, using the hands for support only. Keep lifting with each in-breath and take the chest forward on the out-breath. Keep the hips on the floor and try to feel the curve in the back working down the spine. Hold, breathing steadily and looking ahead. Lower the body slowly to the floor on an out-breath.

Back of neck long

Shoulders rolled back and down

Tailbone tucking under

3 Rest with your head turned to one side on folded arms for a few breaths, then repeat once.

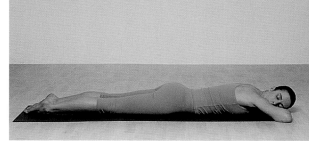

TAKE CARE
• If you have stiff shoulders or a rounded upper spine (kyphosis), try the alternative first (left) and then Snake (see p.318).
• If you have arthritis of the neck, keep the head in line with the spine.

snake

The benefits of this posture are generally the same as for Cobra, but taking the arms back helps with stiffness in the shoulders and the mid-back. Feel the spine lifting away from the floor a vertebra at a time.

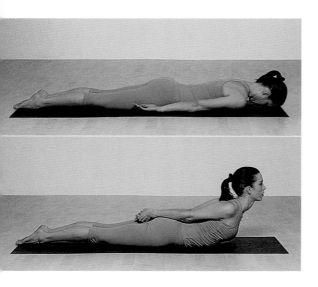

1 Lie on your front with your forehead on the floor and the feet hip-width apart. Have your arms at your sides, palms up. Breathe easily.

2 Rest your arms on your back and interlock the fingers. As you breathe in, lift your head, roll your shoulders back, and stretch the hands toward your feet.

TAKE CARE
• Proceed cautiously if you have back problems.
• If you have neck problems, do not look up.
• Do not hold the posture if you have HBP, heart disease, or a hernia.

3 Use your back muscles to lift yourself higher on the in-breath. Lift your arms away from your back, with your hands still stretching back. Look straight ahead and hold for several breaths, breathing steadily.

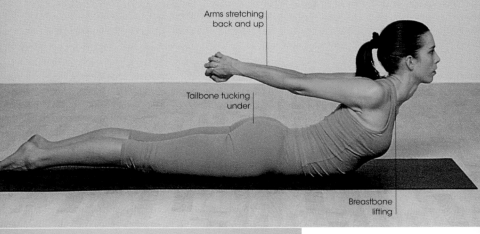

Arms stretching back and up

Tailbone tucking under

Breastbone lifting

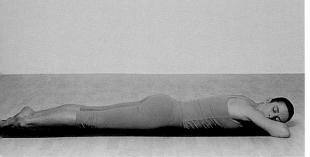

4 Lower yourself slowly to the floor on an out-breath. Relax for a short while with your head turned to one side and resting on your folded arms. Repeat once.

locust

This invigorating posture strengthens the lower back muscles and stretches the front of the body. Be sure to breathe steadily in the final position, and do not strain to lift your legs a long way from the floor.

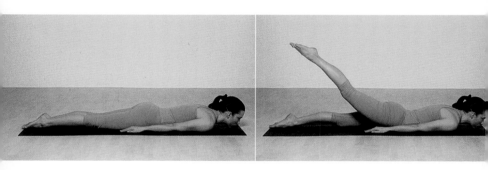

1 Lie on your front with your legs together, your arms by your sides with palms facing down, and your chin on the floor. Take several breaths to prepare yourself.

2 Breathing in, raise your right leg as far as you comfortably can while keeping it straight, keeping your left hip on the floor. Keep the upper body relaxed. Hold for several breaths, then lower on an out-breath. Do on the left and then once more on both sides. (This Step is known as Half Locust.)

TAKE CARE
Stop at Step 2 if you have HBP, heart disease, lower back pain, a peptic ulcer, or a hernia.

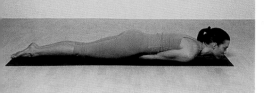

If Half Locust was easy for you, return to the starting position, but this time make fists with your hands and place them under the groin.

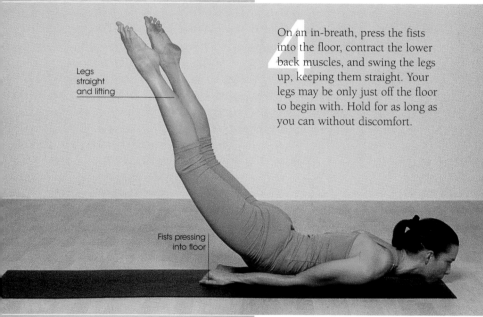

Legs straight and lifting

Fists pressing into floor

On an in-breath, press the fists into the floor, contract the lower back muscles, and swing the legs up, keeping them straight. Your legs may be only just off the floor to begin with. Hold for as long as you can without discomfort.

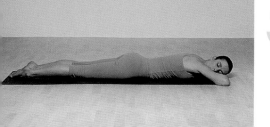

Lower the legs back to the floor on an out-breath and relax with your head turned to one side and resting on your folded arms. Repeat once.

bow

In this pose, the front of the body is stretched like a bow that is about to be fired. It encourages full use of the lungs and has a powerful rejuvenating effect.

1 Lie face down with your legs together and your arms by your sides. Stretch the toes away and relax the shoulders. Take several breaths.

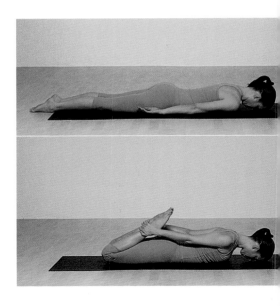

2 Bend your knees to bring your feet toward your hips. Reach back with your arms, one at a time, to hold onto your ankles. (If you cannot reach, loop a belt around each ankle.)

TAKE CARE

If you have HBP, heart disease, a hernia, or back pain, stop at Step 3 and do not hold; avoid altogether if you feel any symptoms.

Keep the arms straight, and as you breathe in, lift your knees and push your feet away from you, bringing your head and shoulders away from the floor at the same time. Pause as you breathe out, then lift the legs a little higher on the in-breath.

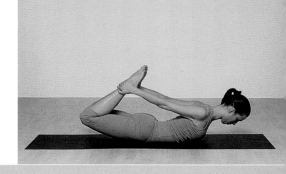

Keep lifting the legs and the upper body on the in-breath to increase the curve through the spine. Feel the body rocking gently to and fro with the breath. If you are very flexible, eventually only the abdomen will be on the floor, but do not strain to achieve this. Stay for several breaths, then lower slowly back to the floor on an out-breath. Release the legs and relax. Repeat once, holding a little longer.

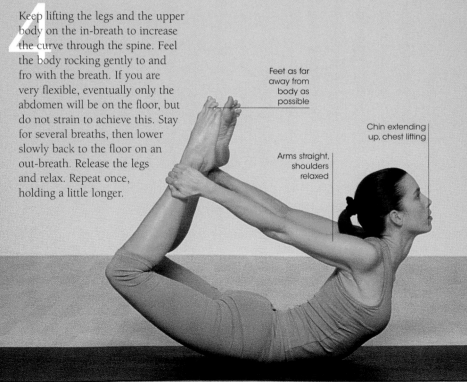

Feet as far away from body as possible

Chin extending up, chest lifting

Arms straight, shoulders relaxed

sun salute

Made up of some of the postures described earlier, this dynamic sequence stimulates and balances your entire body. Once you are able to practice several rounds fluidly, you will feel years younger!

1 Stand with your feet together and bring your palms together in front of your chest. Look straight ahead and take several breaths, lifting up through the body on the in-breath.

2 On an exhalation, open your hands and lower your arms to the side of the body, with the palms facing forward.

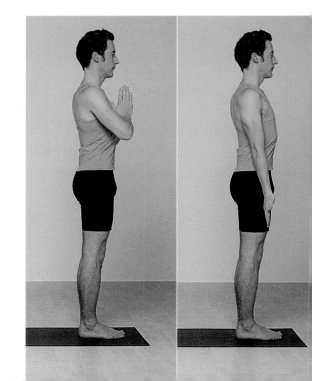

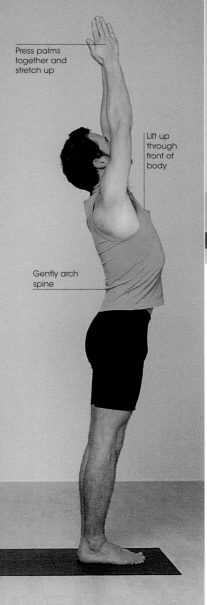

Press palms together and stretch up

Lift up through front of body

Gently arch spine

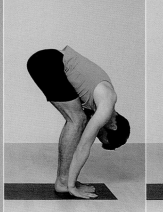

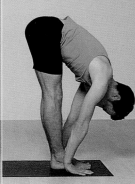

As you breathe in, take the arms out to the side and circle them up to bring the palms together above the head. Look up at the hands and arch the back slightly.

As you exhale, bend the knees and fold forward from the hips, bringing the palms (or the fingertips) to the floor in a relaxed Forward Bend (see p.292).

Breathe in, lengthening through the backs of the legs and the spine, drawing the upper body away from the thighs. Keep your arms as straight as possible. Look at the floor. ▶

6 As you breathe out, bend the knees and take a large step back with the right foot. Keep looking at the floor.

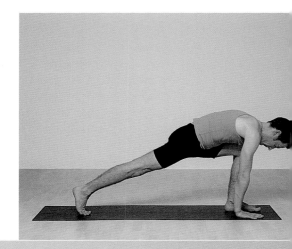

7 As you breathe in, extend through the upper body and look forward to come into Lunge Warrior (see p.300). Push the right heel away from the body.

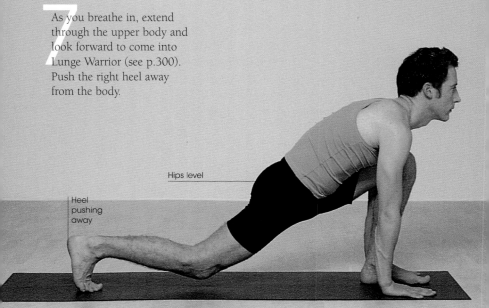

Hips level

Heel pushing away

8 Breathe out as you step back with your left foot to come into Downward Dog (see p.314). Lengthen through your arms, back, and legs. If necessary, keep your knees slightly bent.

9 Holding the breath out, lower your knees and then your upper body to the floor. Stretch your toes back to come onto the front of your feet.

10 Breathing in, come into Cobra (see p.316). Extend through the front of the body, lifting the breastbone forward and up. Roll the shoulders back and down, and look straight ahead. ▶

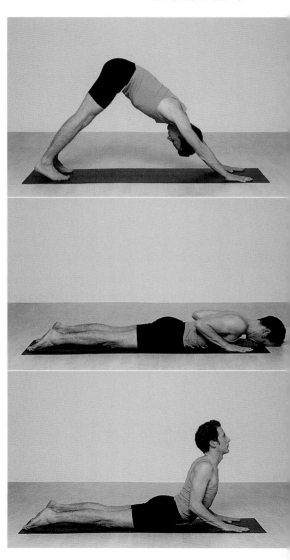

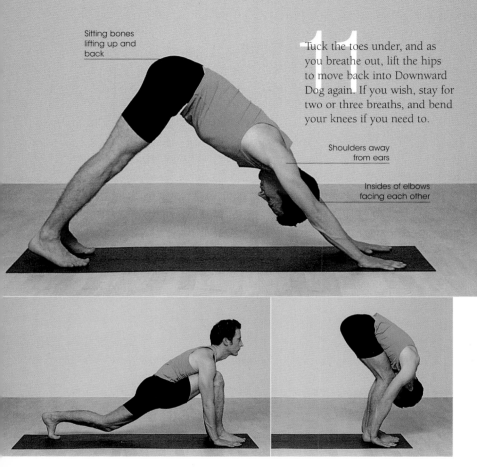

Sitting bones
lifting up and
back

11 Tuck the toes under, and as you breathe out, lift the hips to move back into Downward Dog again. If you wish, stay for two or three breaths, and bend your knees if you need to.

Shoulders away
from ears

Insides of elbows
facing each other

12 As you breathe in, step the right foot forward between the hands to come into Lunge Warrior again. Look straight ahead.

13 Breathe out, bringing your left foot forward to join the right foot, and come into an easy Forward Bend with bent legs. Have the upper body close to the thighs.

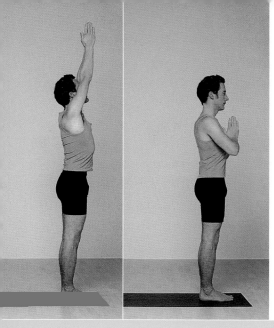

14 As you breathe in, come up, keeping your knees bent and back long, and circling your arms out to the side to bring the palms together above the head. Straighten the legs.

15 As you breathe out, lower your hands to your chest and look straight ahead. Breathe easily. Repeat the entire sequence on the left side to complete one full Sun Salute.

ALTERNATIVES

• Depending on your flexibility, you may find that you need to be on your fingertips, rather than on your palms, for example, when you move back or forward into Lunge Warrior (Steps 7 and 12).
• You may find that you need to keep your back knee on the floor in Lunge Warrior.

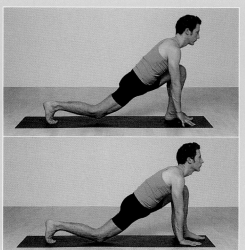

shoulder stand
against a wall

This rejuvenating posture reverses the effects of gravity on the body, and helps bring calm and clarity to the mind. Many people find a folded blanket under the shoulders helps keep the neck free.

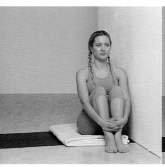
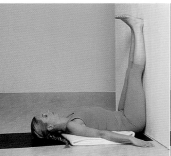
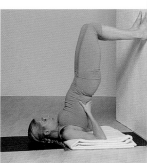

1 Sit sideways against a wall on a folded blanket, 3 ft (1 m) square, with your left hip touching the wall. Breathe easily.

2 Swivel onto your back and stretch the legs up the wall. Your shoulders should be positioned near the edge of the blanket.

3 Bend your knees and push the soles of your feet against the wall to lift yourself up. Support the back with your hands. Your neck is off the blanket.

TAKE CARE
• If you have HBP, a heart condition, a detached retina, glaucoma, neck problems, are very overweight or menstruating, do the alternative (see p.333).
• If you have LBP, come out of any inverted posture very slowly.

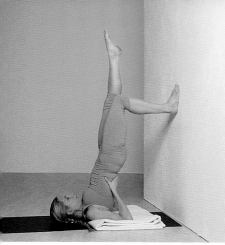

Breathing steadily, keep pushing and lifting to make the back more upright. Make sure the center of the back of the head is on the floor. Lift one leg away from the wall. If you feel any discomfort in the neck or head, do not try to adjust your head, but come down and seek advice from a teacher.

Lift the other leg away to come into Shoulder Stand, supporting your weight on your shoulders and upper arms. Slide your hands higher up your back, press down through the upper arms, and stretch your trunk and legs up. Breathing normally, hold the position for about 30 seconds. You can gradually increase the time that you hold the position as you become more experienced. ▶

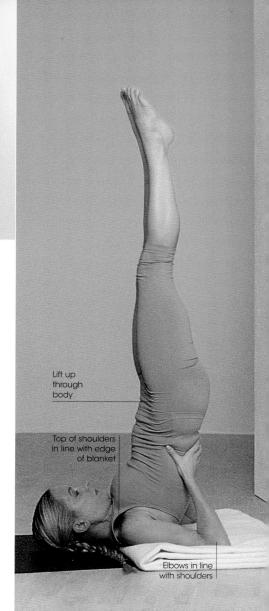

Lift up through body

Top of shoulders in line with edge of blanket

Elbows in line with shoulders

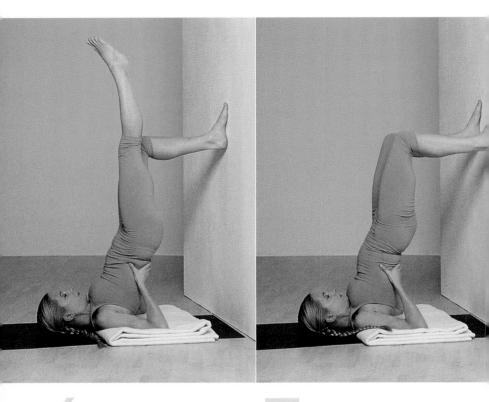

6 To come out of the pose, bend your left knee to bring the sole of your left foot back to the wall. Keep stretching up through the spine and continue to support your back with your hands.

7 Bend your right knee to bring your right foot to the wall. Breathing normally, start to lower your spine slowly to the floor, keeping the back supported as you come down.

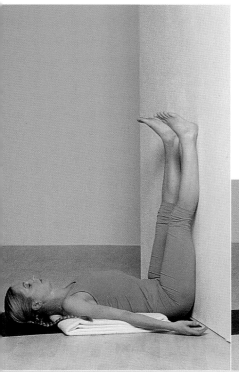

8 When your lower back is on the floor, take your arms out to the side and stay in the position for a few breaths with your legs stretched up the wall.

9 On an out-breath, bend your knees over the chest and roll over onto your side. Stay for a short while before sitting up.

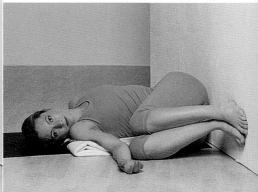

ALTERNATIVE

Lying with your legs up the wall is the only safe inversion if you have HBP, a heart condition, a detached retina, glaucoma, neck problems, or are seriously overweight. It is also advised during menstruation when taking your legs apart can help to relieve tension in the lower abdomen/pelvic region.

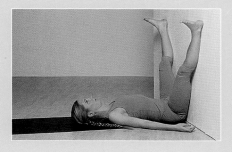

shoulder stand

If you find Shoulder Stand Against a Wall easy, try this version. In the final position, focus on lifting up through the spine and stretching the legs up. Keep relaxed, and breathe smoothly and deeply.

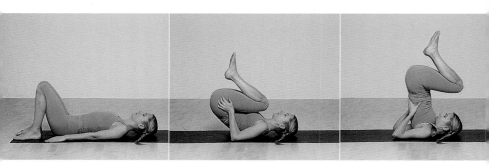

1 Lie on your back with your knees bent and arms by your side, palms down. Make sure the center of the back of the head is on the floor.

2 Inhale, then, bending your knees over your chest, press your arms to the floor and swing your hips up. At the same time, bring your hands up to support your hips. Exhale.

3 Bring your hands on to your back, keeping your upper arms on the floor. Press your hands into the back to bring your weight onto the tops of your shoulders. Make sure your neck is free and relaxed.

TAKE CARE
· As for Shoulder Stand Against a Wall (see p.330).
· A blanket can be helpful, keeping the neck free.

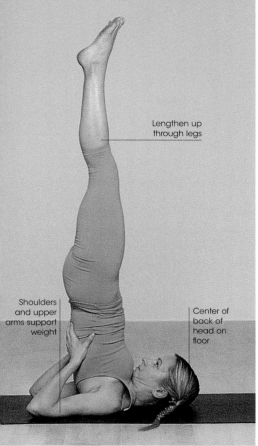

Lengthen up
through legs

Shoulders
and upper
arms support
weight

Center of
back of
head on
floor

4 Pushing your upper arms and elbows into the floor, slide your hands down toward your shoulders to make your upper body vertical. Slowly straighten your legs toward the ceiling and bring the elbows closer together. Breathe easily. Hold the position for a short time only to begin with.

5 On an exhalation, bend the knees toward the head and roll down, supporting yourself with your hands. You may need to let your head and shoulders come off the floor as you roll down.

6 Keep rolling forward to sit up, and relax over the bent knees, as shown here. If you prefer, lie down for a few breaths.

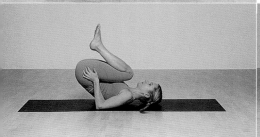

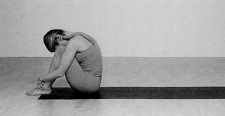

plow

Plow provides a strong forward stretch to the spine and the back of the legs. It can be done on its own, as shown here, or from Shoulder Stand (see p.334). Be careful not to strain the neck.

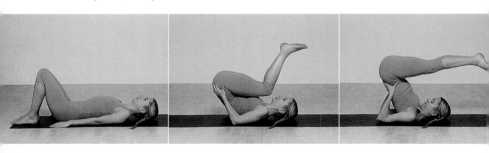

1 Lie on your back with your knees bent and feet hip-width apart. Place the arms at your side, palms facing down. Take several breaths.

2 Inhale; then, bending your knees over your chest, press your arms down on the floor and swing your hips up. Bring your hands up to support your hips, then exhale.

3 Bring your hands onto your back, keeping the upper arms on the floor, as for Shoulder Stand (see p.334). Bring your weight onto the tops of your shoulders, making sure the neck is free and relaxed. Stretch your legs back.

TAKE CARE
- As for Shoulder Stand Against a Wall (see p.330).
- Do not turn your neck from side to side.

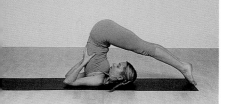

Bring your toes to the floor, while supporting the back with your hands. Keep lifting up through the back and lengthen through the legs.

Tuck your toes under. Stretch your arms out along the floor behind you with the fingers interlocked. Stay in the pose for a short while to begin with, breathing quietly. Then bend the legs and, supporting your back, roll out as for Shoulder Stand (see p.334).

Lift tailbone

Draw elbows together

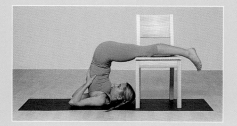

ALTERNATIVES

If you cannot reach the floor with the feet, bend the knees toward your head. Alternatively, have a chair positioned behind your head and let your legs rest on the chair, while supporting your back with your hands.

child

This restorative pose, which develops breath awareness, gently stretches the spine while taking your attention inward. Done as a moving pose, Child strengthens the spinal and abdominal muscles.

1 Kneel and sit back on your heels. Look straight ahead. Place your hands behind your back and hold one wrist with the other hand. Lengthen through the spine. Breathe in.

TAKE CARE

• If you have HBP, glaucoma, a detached retina, or back problems, support your forehead on several blocks or kneel in front of a chair and rest your head on your forearms on the seat.
• Do not move back and forth in the pose if you suffer from epilepsy.

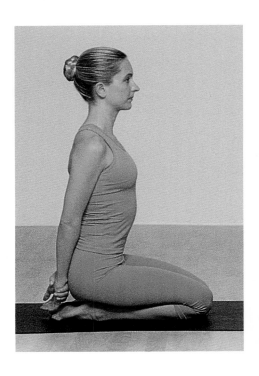

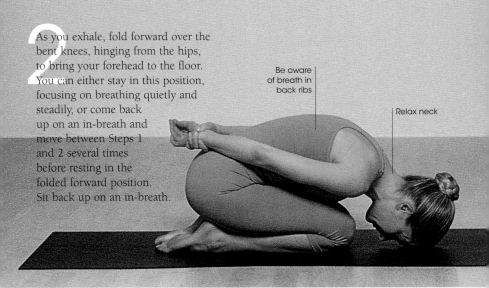

2 As you exhale, fold forward over the bent knees, hinging from the hips, to bring your forehead to the floor. You can either stay in this position, focusing on breathing quietly and steadily, or come back up on an in-breath and move between Steps 1 and 2 several times before resting in the folded forward position. Sit back up on an in-breath.

Be aware of breath in back ribs

Relax neck

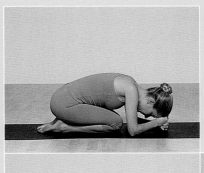

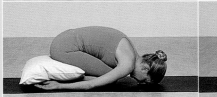

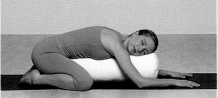

ALTERNATIVES

• If you cannot reach the floor easily with your forehead, support it on your fists, as shown, or on a block.

• If your bottom lifts away from your heels, place a pillow between it and your legs.

• For a very relaxed Child, have your knees apart and lie over a bolster with your head to one side.

sitting stretch
sequence

This simple stretching sequence focuses your attention on the breath. It encourages ribcage breathing, leaving you feeling more alive and alert. Repeat the sequence with the legs crossed the opposite way.

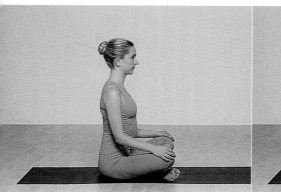 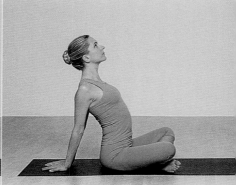

1 Sit cross-legged with your hands resting on your knees. Look straight ahead. Roll the shoulders back and down. Breathe easily.

2 Place your hands behind you, the fingers pointing away from the body. Lean back, lifting the chest. Look slightly upward. Take three full breaths. Come forward again and roll the shoulders back and down.

TAKE CARE
- If you have back problems, omit Step 3 or avoid posture altogether.
- If you have HBP or a heart condition, hold Step 5 for one breath only.

3 Place your hands on the floor in front of you and stretch forward. Slide the hands as far forward as is comfortable for you. Lower your head and take three slow, full breaths.

Lengthen through spine

Hinge forward from hips

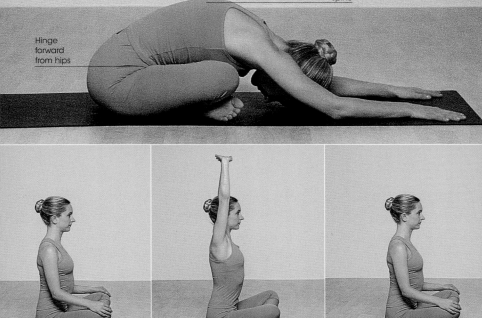

4 Come back up on the in-breath. Bring your hands back to the knees and roll your shoulders back and down again.

5 Interlock your fingers and, breathing in, stretch the arms above your head. Hold for three breaths.

6 Lower the arms. Roll the shoulders back and down, and sit breathing quietly for a while.

sitting twist

This pose encourages spinal flexibility, helps relieve neck and shoulder stiffness, and encourages ribcage breathing. In the final position, look to the side or close your eyes and focus on sensations within the body.

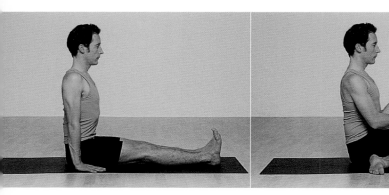

1 Sit with your feet stretched out in front. (If you need to, sit on a block.) Press the hands into the floor and slide your hips back to bring yourself onto the front of your sitting bones. Stretch through the legs.

2 Pull up the right leg and slide your left foot to the outside of your right hip. Place the right foot against the outside of the left thigh. (If this is too difficult, keep the left leg stretched forward.) Pull against the shin to sit up taller.

TAKE CARE

Make sure both sitting bones are on the floor or a block in Step 2.

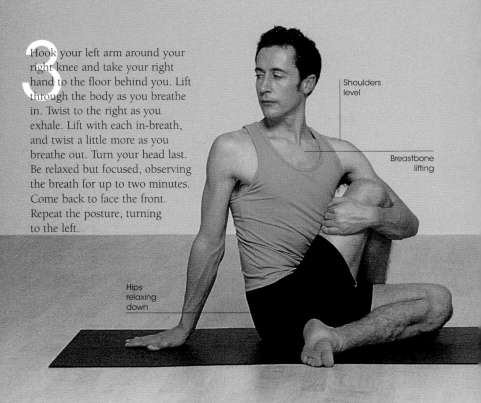

3 Hook your left arm around your right knee and take your right hand to the floor behind you. Lift through the body as you breathe in. Twist to the right as you exhale. Lift with each in-breath, and twist a little more as you breathe out. Turn your head last. Be relaxed but focused, observing the breath for up to two minutes. Come back to face the front. Repeat the posture, turning to the left.

Shoulders level

Breastbone lifting

Hips relaxing down

4 To extend the posture, bring the left arm onto the outside of the right thigh and stretch the fingertips toward the floor as you breathe out.

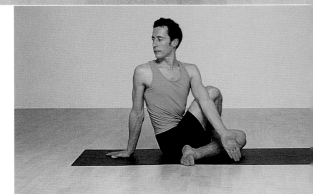

breathing
practices

The following breathing practices will improve your breath awareness and help balance the mind and body. They are particularly useful in helping to quieten the mind for meditation (see p.350).

Breathing practices balance the energy flow within the body, encouraging calm and mental clarity. They also help tone respiratory muscles and keep respiratory passages clear. They are generally practiced after doing some yoga postures or simple stretching exercises. These loosen up the body, releasing any stiffness and tension, and making it easier to be still during the breathing practices. Breath awareness is crucial to learning to observe thoughts, feelings, and patterns of behavior.

Audible breath

Audible breath encourages awareness of the smooth, regular flow of the breath. It is normally practiced sitting and helps quieten the mind, fostering a calm, centered state, helpful for meditation. But it can also be used during posture work to help you stay focused.

To begin the practice, sit comfortably cross-legged or kneeling (see p.261) and breathe through the mouth. Closing the throat slightly, make an "Ahhhh" sound as you breathe in, and a sighing "Haaa" sound as you breathe out.

When you are relaxed doing this, make the same sound in the throat but with your mouth closed. Keep your jaw relaxed. It may help to imagine that you are breathing through a hole in the front of your throat. Breathe easily, focusing on the smooth flow of the breath.

supine abdominal breathing

This practice relaxes the body and the mind, and is good for letting go of tension. Be aware of how easily the breath flows, and feel the calm alertness in the mind once you have completed the practice.

1 Lie on your back with your knees bent and resting against each other, and feet hip-width apart Allow your breath to settle into a smooth, natural rhythm. Become aware of the rise and fall of the abdomen as you breathe. Focus on the out-breath, and allow it to become a little longer than the in-breath.

2 Gradually make the out-breath more complete, by slowly pulling the abdomen back toward the spine as you exhale. As you inhale, let the abdomen swell out. Repeat several times. Then, each time you exhale, pull up the pelvic floor tightly (as if stopping yourself from urinating).

3 As you breathe in, keep the abdomen and pelvic floor slightly contracted, and gently reinforce the contractions as you breathe out. Feel the in-breath in the ribcage. Take several breaths like this, then relax the abdomen and pelvic floor and let the breath be completely free. It should feel quiet and relaxed.

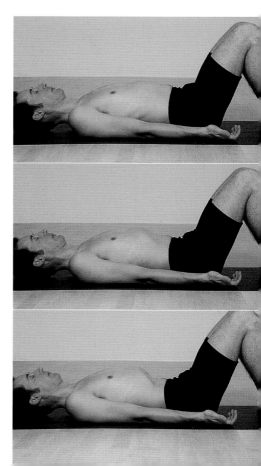

mock inhalation

This practice increases awareness of the diaphragm in breathing, and increases its strength and flexibility. The quality of the breath after the practice makes it a great way to start the day and to prepare for meditation. It involves making a full exhalation, and then closing the throat (as if you were holding your breath) and expanding the ribs as if breathing in – a "mock inhalation." Practice in the lying position first. If the first in-breath after the practice feels rushed, try a smaller "mock inhalation" at Step 3. The technique is simple, but a teacher can help you make sure you get it right. Seek advice if you have any problems.

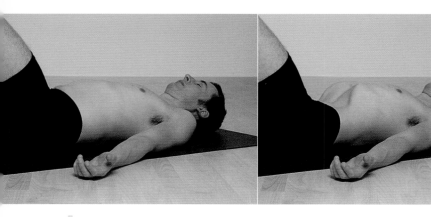

1 Lie on the floor with your knees bent, arms away from the side of the body, and palms facing up. Close the eyes and allow the breath to settle into a natural, regular rhythm.

2 Allow the breath to become deeper and make the out-breath longer. Breathe in fully, expanding the rib cage and letting the abdomen swell. Exhale completely, pulling the abdomen in fully.

TAKE CARE
• Avoid the practice if you have HBP or active inflammation or bleeding in the abdominal region.
• This practice is best avoided during menstruation because it creates strong negative pressures in the abdomen.

ALTERNATIVE
Stand with your legs about hip-width apart and your knees slightly bent. Lean forward a little way, rounding the back slightly. Rest your hands lightly on your thighs, your elbows out to the side. Follow Steps 2 to 4 below.

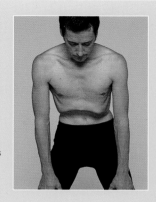

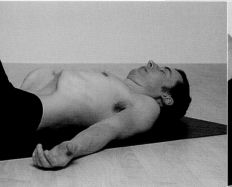

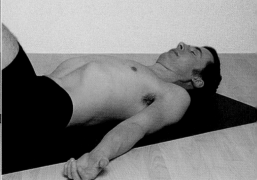

3 Holding your breath out, relax the abdomen. Simultaneously, expand the chest, without breathing in, to suck the abdomen in and up, forming a hollow at the base of the ribs. Hold until you feel the natural impulse to breathe in.

4 To breathe in, relax the ribs, open the throat, and, contracting the abdomen slightly, allow the breath to flow in smoothly. Repeat twice more, breathing normally for about 20 seconds between each round.

alternate nostril breathing

This practice balances the flow of energy within you. Practice the technique shown below, then try this. Take three breaths through the left nostril, then three through the right. Then breathe in through the left and out through the right for three breaths. Next breathe in through the right and out through the left for three breaths. Then take three breaths through both nostrils, focusing your awareness of the breath on the point between your eyebrows. Finally, sit quietly, letting the breath flow freely.

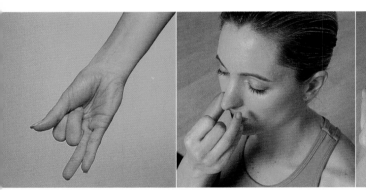
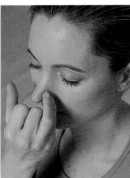

1 Fold in the first two fingers of the right hand, as shown. The thumb is used to close the right nostril, the ring finger to close the left. Press gently against the side of the nose.

2 Start by breathing through the left nostril, closing the right with the thumb. The breath should be smooth and quiet with a natural pause between the in-breath and the out-breath.

3 To switch to the right nostril, first close the left with the ring finger, then release the thumb. To breathe through the left again, first close the right, then open the left. Practice switching from side to side.

cooling breath

Breathing through the nostrils is emphasized in yoga, but in Cooling Breath you breathe in through the mouth. As you suck in the air, it makes a hissing sound and produces an "icy" cooling effect in the mouth. This provides a focus for your awareness, and calms the body and the mind. At the end of the in-breath, close your mouth and exhale through both nostrils. The practice is very beneficial when you are overheating physically or emotionally. There are two ways of positioning the tongue, as described below.

TAKE CARE

• As the incoming air is not filtered by the nose in Cooling Breath, practice only where the air quality is good.
• Avoid this practice if you have asthma or other respiratory conditions, or sensitive teeth.

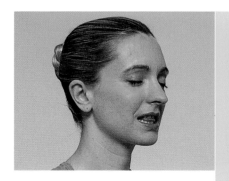

Have your teeth slightly apart and the tongue between them. With eyes closed, slowly suck the air in. It will make a hissing noise, and cool the tongue and roof of the mouth.

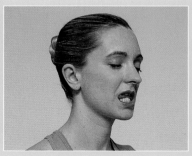

ALTERNATIVE

In this version, the tongue is folded up against the roof of the mouth. Breathe in slowly and deeply through the teeth. You will be able to feel the coolness on the tongue, gums, and roof of the mouth.

meditation

Regular meditation has great restorative powers, helping bring your energies into balance. It helps to keep your mind clear throughout the day and can aid sleep at night when previously it was elusive.

Sit in a comfortable but alert way. Scan the body, letting go of any tension you are holding (in your face, neck, shoulders, upper body, hips, legs, and feet). Close your eyes and let your breath settle into an easy, regular rhythm. Do not try actively to shut out sounds and other sensations; just let them be there and let your senses withdraw from them as you focus on your breath. Be aware of the coolness of the air at the tip of the nostril as you breathe in and the warmth of the air there as you exhale.

To begin with, thoughts will inevitably arise and sensations will distract you. You cannot force the mind to be empty, but do not let yourself react to these disturbances. Observe them objectively as they come into the mind and let them go as you continue to focus on the breath. Do not let yourself be carried away on a train of thought.

If you find focusing on the breath difficult, use the simple mantra "So Ham." "So Ham" means "I am That" (the universal life force). Silently say "So" as you breathe in and "Ham" as you breathe out.

PRACTICAL MATTERS
• Choose a time when you can remain undisturbed for at least 15 minutes.
• Choose a room (or space outdoors) that is quiet, uncluttered, and not cold.
• Choose a posture – sitting or kneeling on the floor or sitting in a chair – that you will be able to sustain easily for some time.

Eventually, if you practice meditation regularly, you may find that you can dispense with the focus on the breath or the mantra, and just sit quietly but alertly, observing the stillness and the feeling of space. You will be able to let yourself "be" in the present moment, with no thought of the future or the past.

If you can find this quiet, peaceful state, you may like to ask yourself the following three questions:

"Who is the 'I' that is observing this stillness?"

"What is the nature of the 'I' that is observing this stillness?"

"Where is the 'I' that is observing this stillness?"

Do not try to answer the questions, just let your awareness answer for you. You may come to realize that the "I" that is observing is not your ego but simply a "center of consciousness," or limitless energy.

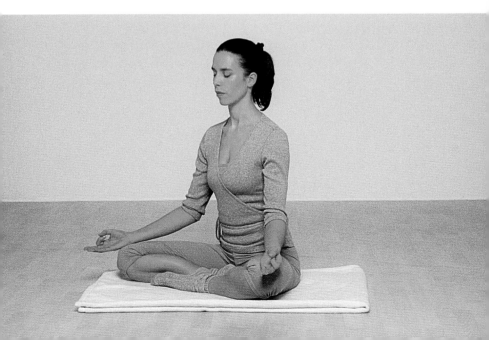

relaxation

Relaxing at the end of a yoga session gives the body and mind a chance to absorb the benefits of your practice. More generally, relaxation techniques can be used anywhere, anytime, to "let go."

Progressive relaxation

Lying down is the best position for relaxation because it provides the greatest relief for the spine from the pressure of gravity. Try this practice after a yoga session, or whenever you have 10 to 20 minutes to spare. Wear warm clothes and/or cover yourself with a blanket. Try recording this guided relaxation, or ask a friend to read it to you slowly.

Lie with your knees bent, feet hip-width apart, arms away from your body, and backs of hands on the floor. Have the center of the back of your head on the floor. (If your neck is uncomfortable in this position, place a block or pillow under your head.) Stretch through your arms to your fingertips, then let the arms and

shoulders relax. Unless you have a back problem, stretch your legs out. Flex your toes toward you, then let go, so that the feet and legs relax outward. Be aware of your surroundings, then close your eyes.

Be aware of the back of your head and let it sink down. Let your eyes feel heavy beneath the eyelids. Relax your jaw so the teeth part slightly. Smile a little to relax your face. Swallow and let your neck relax. Relax your right hand and arm, your right shoulder, the right side of your trunk. Relax your right hip and buttock, your right leg and foot. Then do the same on the left: hand and arm, shoulder, left side of trunk, left hip, buttock, leg, and foot. Feel that your body is now relaxed from your waist to your feet, from your chest to your feet, from the top of your head to your feet.

Become aware of your breath. Observe it entering and leaving the body. As you breathe in, the chest and abdomen gently rise; as you breathe out they sink back down. Be aware of a sensation of expansion and lightness as you breathe in, of letting go as you breathe out. Then, just be aware of breathing out and letting go. Enjoy the quiet and calm.

When you are ready, become aware again of the ground beneath you, the touch of the air on your skin. Be aware of sounds outside the room, then inside. Gently move your fingers and toes. Take one or two deeper breaths, then stretch and yawn or sigh. Turn onto your right side. Stay for a few breaths with your eyes closed, then slowly sit up. Open your eyes.

Instant relaxation

If lying down is not possible or time is short, try the following: Squeeze your eyes tightly, clench your teeth, tense your shoulders, clench your fists and buttocks, tense your legs and clench your toes. Hold your whole body as tightly as possible for a count of three, then let go completely. Repeat twice. Then breathe easily.

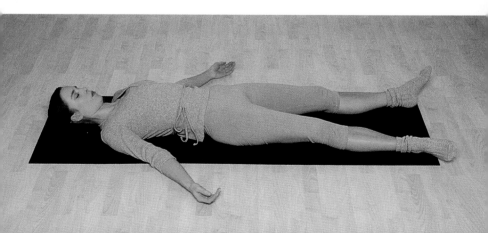

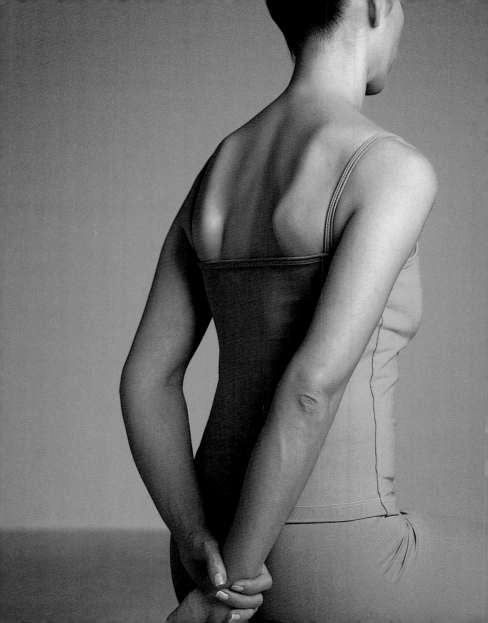

programs

Here are seven programs to help you feel young and more alive. Remember to centre yourself and do some preliminary stretches first, and to relax afterward. Maximize the benefits with breathing and meditation, and adjust your lifestyle if you need to.

① strong
heart & lungs

These postures will help stretch and strengthen muscles used in breathing, and strengthen your heart. Focus on breathing deeply and evenly in the postures. Improve your breath awareness with breathing basics (see p.268) and breathing practices (see p.344), and increase your aerobic endurance with the Sun Salute (see p.324).

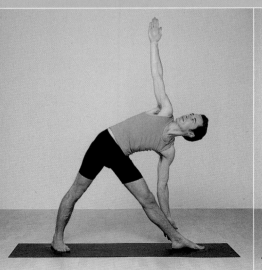

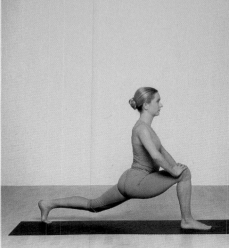

① **Triangle** (see pp.296–297)

② **Lunge Warrior** (see pp.300–301)

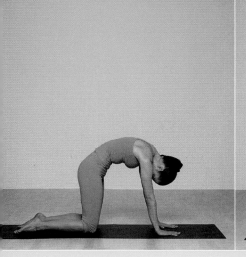

3 Cat (see pp.308–309)

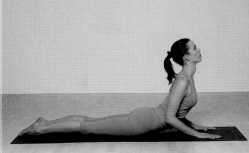

4 Cobra (see pp.316–317)

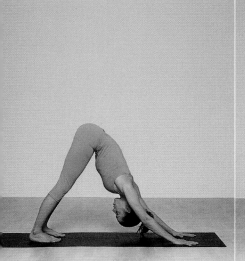

5 Downward Dog (see pp.314–315)

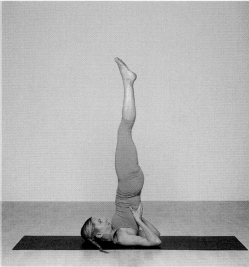

6 Shoulder Stand (see pp.334–335)

② digestive system
energizer

Here are six postures that together will stretch, massage, and relax your abdominal muscles, bringing energy to the digestive system. Complement them with mock inhalation (see p.346), abdominal breathing (see p.345), and relaxation (see p.352). A balanced diet and eating calmly will help maximize the benefits of the program.

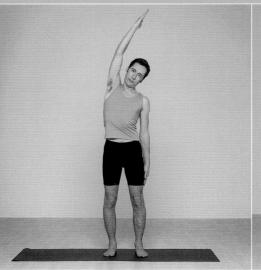

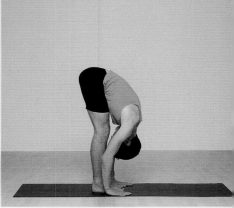

❶ **Standing Side Stretch** (see pp.286–287)

❷ **Forward Bend** (see pp.292–293)

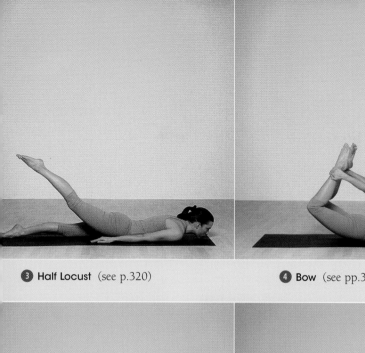

3 Half Locust (see p.320)

4 Bow (see pp.322–323)

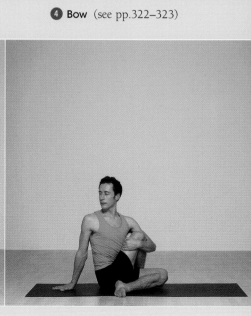

5 Child (see pp.338–339)

6 Sitting Twist (see pp.342–343)

3 develop a
healthy spine

This program encourages spinal alignment and flexibility, strengthens postural muscles, and improves blood supply to the spinal region. Complement it with the Sun Salute (see p.324), supine abdominal breathing (see p.345), and relaxation (see p.352). Develop your postural awareness throughout the day, and be positive.

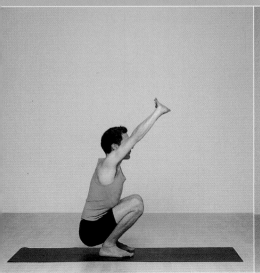

1 **Full Squat** (see pp.290–291)

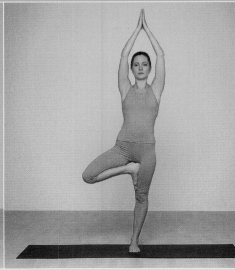

2 **Tree** (see pp.302–303)

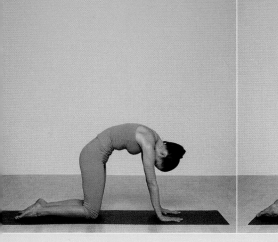

3 Cat (see pp.308–309)

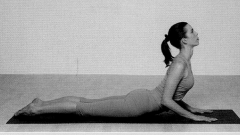

4 Cobra (see pp.316–317)

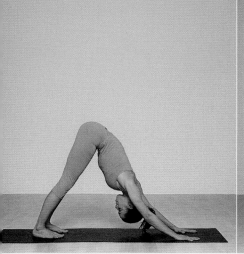

5 Downward Dog (see pp.314–315)

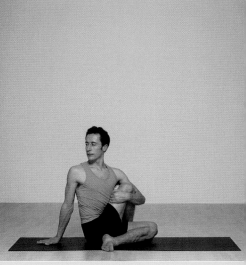

6 Sitting Twist (see pp.342–343)

4 for balance & concentration

Complete the postures shown on these two pages to keep your brain relaxed but alert. Focus on keeping the body and the mind as still as possible while you practise. Keep your breath slow and even throughout. Complement the program with alternate nostril breathing (see p.348) and meditation (see p.350).

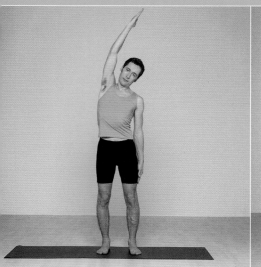

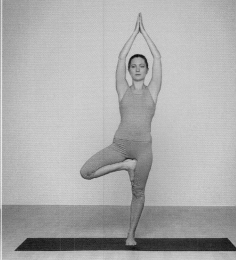

1 Standing Side Stretch (see pp.286–287)

2 Tree (see pp.302–303)

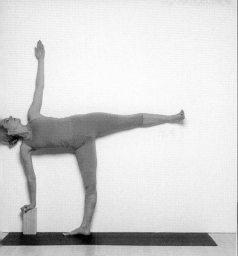

3 **Half Moon** (see pp.304–305)

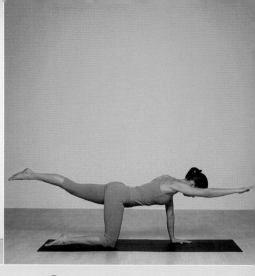

4 **Cat Balance** (see pp.310–311)

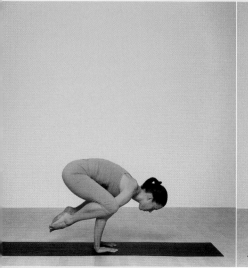

5 **Crow** (see pp.306–307)

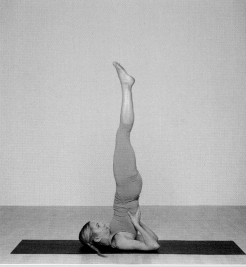

6 **Shoulder Stand** (see pp.334–335)

⑤ to ease
menopause

Warrior and Locust are energizing postures, Half Moon helps relieve pelvic congestion and encourages balance, while Shoulder Stand is rejuvenating and may help hot flushes. Downward Dog and Child are calming. Complement these postures with breathing practices (see p.348), meditation (see p.350), a healthy lifestyle, and adequate rest.

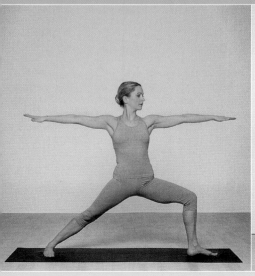

❶ Side Warrior (see pp.298–299)

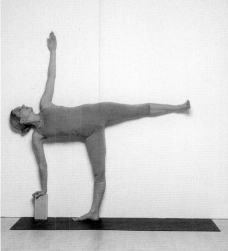

❷ Half Moon (see pp.304–305)

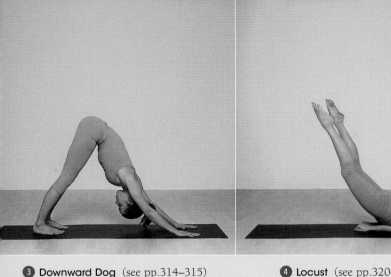

3 Downward Dog (see pp.314–315)

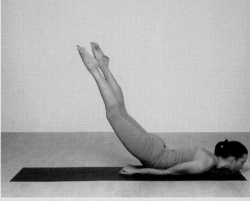

4 Locust (see pp.320–321)

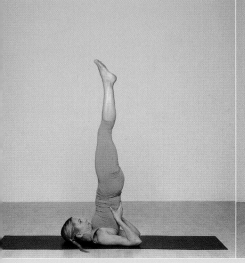

5 Shoulder Stand (see pp.334–335)

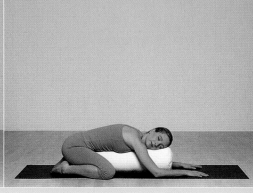

6 Child (see pp.338–339)

6 releasing hips & shoulders

If your day involves long hours standing or sitting hunched over a desk or steering wheel, try these postures to help loosen the hips and shoulders, and ease discomfort. Start the program with some preliminary stretches (see p. 270) and end with the progressive relaxation practice (see p.352) to help make it even more effective.

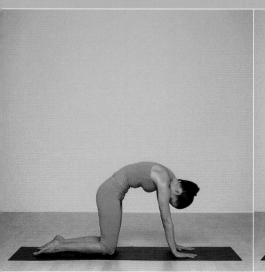

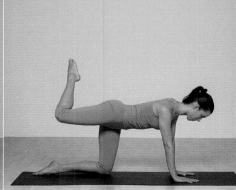

1 Cat (see pp.308–309)

2 Cat Circles (see pp.312–313)

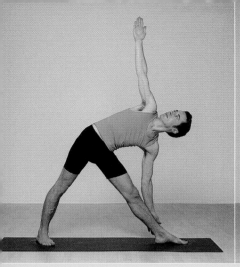

3 **Triangle** (see pp.296–297)

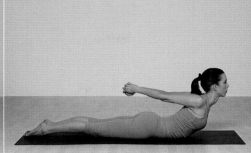

4 **Snake** (see pp.318–319)

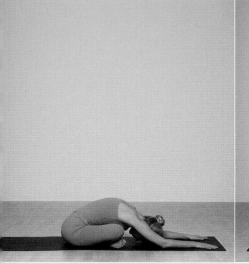

5 **Sitting Stretch Sequence** (see pp.340–341)

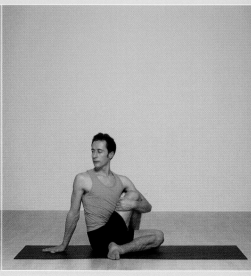

6 **Sitting Twist** (see pp.342–343)

7 boost your
immunity

Keeping your vitality depends on a healthy immune system, which benefits from moderate exercise and regular sleep. This program can help bring energy to the immune system. Complement it with sectional breathing (see p.269), alternate nostril breathing (see p.348), and progressive relaxation (see p.352).

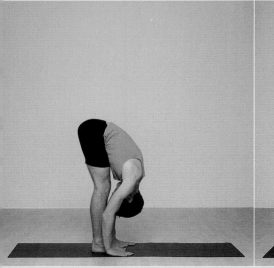

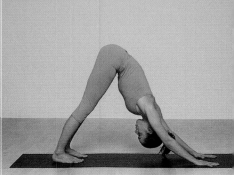

1 Forward Bend (see pp.292–293)

2 Downward Dog (see pp.314–315)

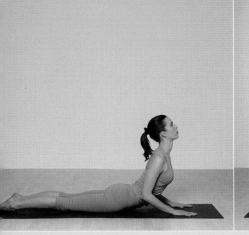
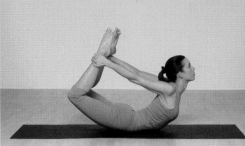

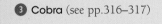
3 **Cobra** (see pp.316–317)

4 **Bow** (see pp.322–333)

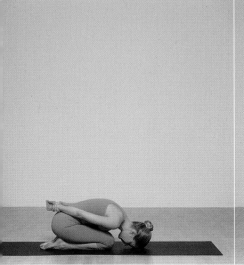
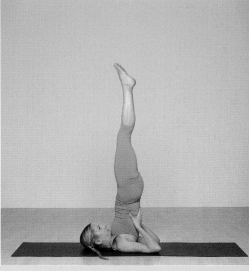

5 **Child** (see pp.338–339)

6 **Shoulder Stand** (see pp.334–335)

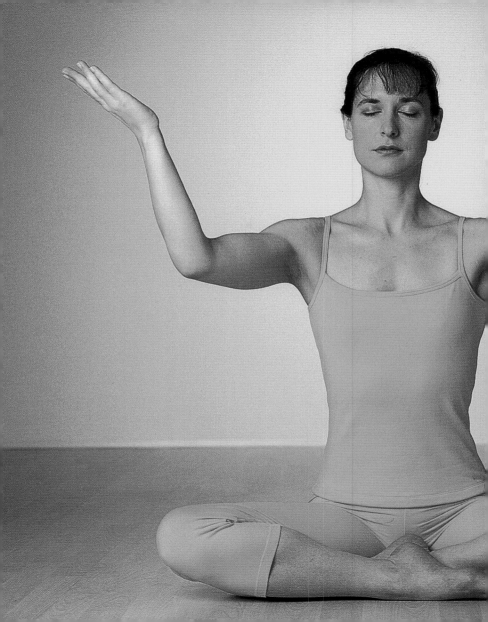

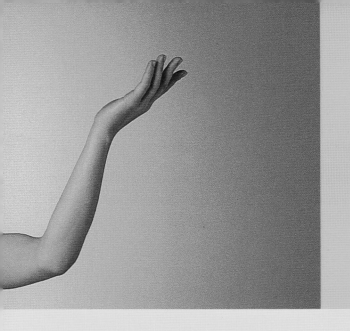

confident

feeling
confident

To practise yoga is to develop self-awareness on a physical, mental, and emotional level. Such awareness offers liberation from low self-esteem and a firm foundation on which to build self-confidence.

Practising yoga gives you the time and the techniques to become aware of aspects of yourself that you tend to overlook in everyday life. At a physical level, yoga teaches you to be aware of your breathing patterns, and of areas of tension or tiredness in your muscles and joints. At a mental and emotional level, yoga helps you to notice your patterns of thought, to be aware of the effects of your attitudes and habits, and to understand your worries and concerns. Yoga is a practical tool that helps you to become self-aware.

This self-awareness is the basis of self-respect. When you begin to respect yourself, you start to build your self-confidence. Yoga nourishes and strengthens the body, mind, and spirit. In practising it regularly, you will become more aware of your real needs, and grow to recognize your own abilities, attitudes, preferences,

HEALTH CONCERNS

If a health practitioner has advised you not to over-exert yourself physically, or if you have any other health concerns, seek advice from a qualified yoga therapist or teacher (see p.495) before using this book. Page 9 provides basic advice for some common medical conditions and, where appropriate, "Take Care" advice and "Alternatives" are given for individual practices. If you are pregnant, or have recently given birth, ask a suitably qualified yoga teacher which practices would be appropriate for you.

and habits. Yoga promotes confidence and assuredness, enabling you to be comfortable and at ease with yourself. It gives unlimited access to the relaxed and respectful understanding that underpins self-confidence.

Unlike some forms of exercise, yoga is suitable for everyone. Whatever your age or level of fitness, yoga is a very safe form of exercise, provided you work within your limits. However, please read through the text in the box below-left, entitled "Health Concerns," before you begin, as some yoga practices can be physically demanding.

Causes of low self-esteem

All too often the erosion of confidence and self-esteem begins with unfavorable comparisons with other people or with an idealized, unrealistic notion of who you think you are or ought to be. Then the spiral of self-criticism and self-recrimination begins, and you lose touch with the reality of your own strengths and weaknesses. You build for yourself a punishing self-image based on harsh expectations.

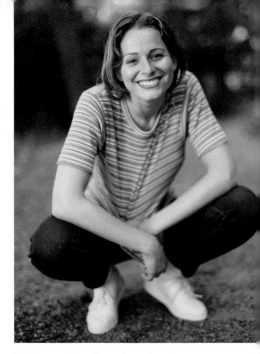

Vitality, good health, and emotional wellbeing are all rooted in the easeful self-confidence which yoga practice develops.

You may come to feel permanently anxious and dissatisfied: everything you do or say, even the way you sleep and eat, does not feel good enough. This is a debilitating burden to carry around with you everywhere, and although your lack of confidence may be psychological and emotional, it can manifest its heaviness in many physical symptoms.

DEALING WITH OTHER PEOPLE'S BEHAVIOR

Sometimes it may appear that the cause of poor self-confidence is another person or the relationship that you have with another person. It is true that there are certain individuals in whose company you may feel buoyant and confident, and others whose very presence makes you feel nervous and inadequate. But this is not to say that other people hold the key to your own self-confidence. You must find your own inner ease and balance, so that you can meet with equilibrium whatever responses you receive in daily life.

If you are involved in relationships with people who persistently seem to make you feel bad about yourself, you owe it to yourself to explore the reasons for this. It may be that you cannot practically avoid dealing with these people, and so you need to learn how to return always to your sense of inner strength and balance in your interactions with them. It may be also that you need to find ways to end relationships that are truly harmful, or in which the power imbalances are severely damaging. While yoga is a valuable help during such change, you may also need the support of a counselor or therapist to address these issues.

For example, you may begin to assume poor sitting or standing postures, or you may be uncomfortable when you lie down to rest. If your body remains in a state of constant discomfort and tension for long enough, your self-confidence can become further eroded, blocking energy and making you tired, irritable, and cross with yourself.

Low energy levels can also be related to poor nutrition and inadequate breathing. Poor breathing habits can also make it hard to maintain concentration. A distracted mind is characterized by an inability to remain in the present and can become full of self-deprecatory fears and self-accusatory anxieties that may be projected into the future. These kinds of thoughts are every bit as dangerous to self-esteem as the tyrant of negative self-image.

There are a number of lifestyle habits that can erode self-esteem. Over-consumption of caffeine can reduce your ability to concentrate and impair your sleep, leading to self-criticism and depression. The use of nicotine, alcohol, marijuana, and other recreational drugs can make it difficult to be honest with yourself, and without real honesty there can be no firm ground for self-confidence. It is worth investigating the rhythms and patterns of your daily life to check for unnecessary and avoidable items of conflict, stress, and energy depletion that can diminish your sense of self-worth. For example, maybe that exhausting daily 10- minute ride in a bus crammed with bad-tempered commuters could be more productively replaced with an enjoyable 30-minute walk?

How yoga can help

Kindness is the best first aid for a wounded self-image. Compassionate awareness gives you freedom from the dictates of negative self-image because it helps you to recognize what really is the best and most comfortable way for you to be. By consistent repetition of some simple yoga practices, you can effectively reinforce the habit of kindly self-awareness that will eventually eradicate the root causes of self-recrimination and poor self-esteem.

The yoga practices in this book all use breath as a way to understand and develop the interaction between body, mind, and emotions. The practices teach how the focus of your mind can alter your breath, and how the change in the breath can help you to communicate more intelligently with your body. Once the body begins to respond, you enter a "positive feedback loop": the sense of wellbeing that you experience physically has a profound impact on your emotional and mental states. These in turn influence your breath, which promotes a further deepening into ease with the physical body, which makes you feel even better about yourself.

It is an expanding spiral of joy that is deeply practical and very simple. It works to counter the downward spirals of depression and poor self-image, and creates an openhearted ease of confidence and positive self-image that is transformatory. Others notice the positive benefits of your yoga practice and are more positive in their behavior to you, affirming your transformation from without.

The four essential qualities

The yoga practices in this section are designed to promote ease, develop balance, build strength, and sharpen focus. They work with the physical body and breath to access the calm confidence that comes from a more gentle way of living.

Promoting ease

At the heart of a healthy sense of self-confidence is an ease with yourself, a sense of compassion for who you are. To mobilize the energy and strength that comes from developing balance, strength, and focus, you need to establish a comforting confidence in understanding who you are.

Above all, the practice of Full Yogic Breath promotes ease. It helps you to unlearn poor breathing habits and allows you to take full advantage of the lungs' capacity to draw in vitality and confidence with every breath. When you use this practice in your yogic poses, you release farther and deeper into the work of self-transformation and build stronger foundations for self-esteem. When you focus on the exhalation in the

Humming Breath, you tell yourself you can be easeful and relaxed with who you are. Resting in this ease is the time to let destructive habits and self-criticism pass away, and to use the sound vibrations to nurture and nourish the newly emerging, confident, and powerful self. The relaxation poses – Corpse and Reverse Corpse – together with Resting Crocodile and Hare all teach you about surrender and easeful rest in the moment.

Developing balance

Without steady balance there is no firm ground on which to develop a sense of self-worth. When you have balance, you can be still or move with poise, reflecting a balanced state of mind and emotions.

You can work toward mental and emotional equanimity by developing coordinated balance in the physical body, by linking the breath with the body, and by learning to maintain physical poise in positions that you would not have to do in everyday life (for example, when you stand on your head or shoulders). When you develop balance in your body through yoga, you are better able to withstand the challenges and difficulties of life.

Alternate Nostril Breath, Psychic Triangle Breath, and the Breath Balancing pose all teach how to become self-observant, attentive, and patient as you notice a slow but steady change. These practices develop wonder and compassion, for every inhalation and every exhalation links us to the source of life, and to the potential for unbounded confidence, power, and trust.

The more physically demanding balances such as Headstand, Tree, and Dancer require and promote clarity of purpose and perseverance. It takes consistent repetition to master

YOGA PRACTICES FOR THE FOUR QUALITIES

The four qualities of ease, balance, strength, and focus together will help you develop self-confidence. The key postures promoting each quality are listed below. An easeful and balanced foundation is the basis for strength and focus.

Ease
Corpse (see p.381)
Full Yogic Breath (see p.387)
Resting Crocodile (see p.418)
Hare (see p.438)
Spinal Twist & Spinal Twist 2 (see p.454, 456)
Humming Breath (see p.462)

Balance
Yogic Rock and Roll (see p.393)
Tree (see p.404)
Dancer (see p.406)
Snake (see p.416)
Camel (see p.432)
Headstand (see p.450)
Alternate Nostril Breathing (see p.459)
Psychic Triangle Breath (see p.458)
Breath Balancing (see p.463)

Strength
Stirring the Pot (see p.396)
Triangle (see p.402)
Boat (see p.408)
Stoking the Fire (see p.460)
Shining the Skull (see p.461)
Invocation of Energy (see p.464)

Focus
Bow and Arrow (see p.400)
Thunderbolt (see p.426)
Philosopher (see p.428)
Roaring Lion (see p.430)
Concentrated Gazing (see p.466)
Gesture of Consciousness (see p.468)
Gesture of Knowledge (see p.469)
Inner Silence Meditation (see p.470)
Deep Relaxation (see p.472)

these postures, but in practicing them, you develop the clarity of focus to see through negative self-image, and build the perseverance necessary to grow surely in self-confidence.

Building strength

The power to remain poised and balanced in self-esteem requires strength. The strength to remain balanced is a supple strength that enables you to adapt to situations while retaining the power to stand

your ground if necessary. The core of physical strength is in the abdomen: the abdominal muscles support the work of the back muscles to hold you upright, and the "fire in your belly" generates the energy for you to accomplish what you need to do.

The most effective yogic practices for developing abdominal strength are the breathing practices Shining the Skull and Stoking the Fire. Combined with Boat, Triangle, and Stirring the Pot, they enable you to develop a core of strength that is truly empowering. When you then practice the Invocation of Energy, you can understand that the world is full of powerful energy available to give, take, and share with each other.

Sharpening focus

Clarity of focus is crucial to self-esteem. To feel confident in yourself you need to be able to focus both within and without. Internal focus is necessary to understand clearly your

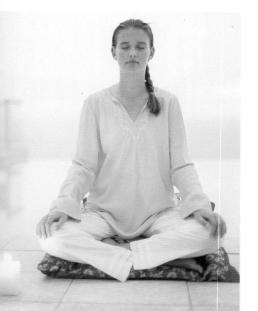

As you develop physical strength and balance, you acquire the emotional equilibrium to feel truly confident.

strengths and weaknesses, and to be compassionate about yourself. External focus is necessary so that you can respond effectively to the situations in which you find yourself, whatever they may be.

Using the focus of the eye in yoga postures helps to sharpen the focus of the mind's eye, to develop clarity of purpose that is at the heart of self-confidence. It is the practice of Concentrated Gazing that most simply and directly teaches the single-pointed gaze. Although, for the most part, the focus of the gaze is an external object, for some of the time the eyes are closed, allowing the inner eye to develop its capacities, too. The Inner Silence Meditation develops this capacity still further, strengthening the concentration of your attention.

The elegant sitting poses – Thunderbolt and Philosopher – provide a physical expression for the focusing of attention, while the simple mudras, or hand gestures, provide subtle but profound physical signs that give further encouragement for the settling of the mind into concentrated awareness.

HOW TO USE THIS SECTION

Confident is divided into three sub-sections. **Foundations** provides guidance on doing yoga and some basic breathing and preliminary stretches. Familiarize yourself with them first before moving on to **Building Blocks**. This contains a selection of postures and breathing practices, as well as a simple meditation and relaxation technique. Work through these postures gradually, selecting one or two to work on at a time, rather than trying to do them all at once. Look at the photographs first to get a feel for the overall shape of the posture. Then follow the accompanying step-by-step instructions carefully. If you find a posture difficult to do, work on the preliminary steps first or try the alternative, if one is given.

Programs combines selected postures and other practices in a series of short yoga programs designed for particular situations and needs. Make sure that you understand how to do the postures first before trying these programs.

Yoga is traditionally learned from a teacher, and you will benefit from going to a class, if you are not already doing so. Organizations that can help you find a qualified teacher are listed on page 495.

the basics

In yoga, basic standing, sitting, and lying-down positions are important in their own right, helping you develop stability and awareness of the benefits of alignment for your posture and breathing, and for the free flow of energy. They also provide the foundations on which other postures are developed.

In addition, being able to sit comfortably and steadily is important for breathing practices and also for meditation, helping you remain focused without distractions from physical tensions. Lying down is often used to develop body and breath awareness, and to relax and allow

your body to absorb the beneficial effects of other yoga practices.

If you find it impossible to achieve the full posture, it can be very helpful to use a prop, such as a block or cushion, to make sure you do not strain your body.

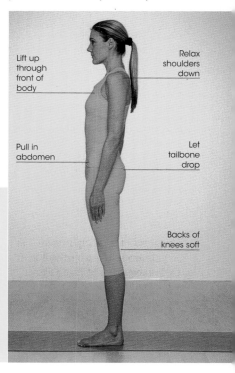

Lift up through front of body

Relax shoulders down

Pull in abdomen

Let tailbone drop

Backs of knees soft

STANDING
Stand up straight with your feet parallel, hip-width apart, and your ears, tops of shoulders, hips, and ankles in line. Press your feet into the ground and lift up through your body. Broaden across the top of the chest. Feel balanced in all directions, your head as if suspended by a thread from the ceiling. Look straight ahead, relax, and breathe easily.

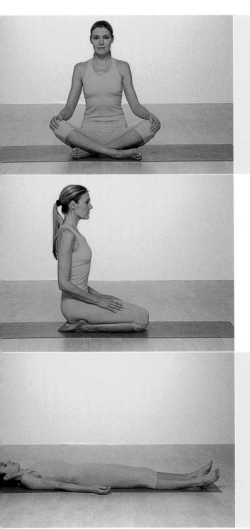

EASY SITTING

This basic posture is good for breathing practices. Cross your shins with the feet under the opposite knee. Position yourself on the front edge of your sitting bones, with the spine long and the head erect. Allow the hips to relax. If your knees are higher than your hips, sit on a block or another support.

KNEELING

Try this position if you find basic cross-legged sitting uncomfortable. Sit on your heels with the tops of your thighs facing the ceiling. Alternatively, if you are going to stay longer, position your knees and feet hip-width apart and sit on blocks, a folded blanket, or a bolster. Keep your spine long and head erect. Rest your hands on your thighs or in your lap.

LYING

Lie on your back to relax at the end of a session or between postures. Lie with your legs stretched out, hip-width apart, feet and legs relaxing out, arms away from your sides, and backs of the hands on the floor. Rest the center of the back of the head on the floor. If you feel any discomfort in your lower back, bend your knees. This is known as Corpse pose.

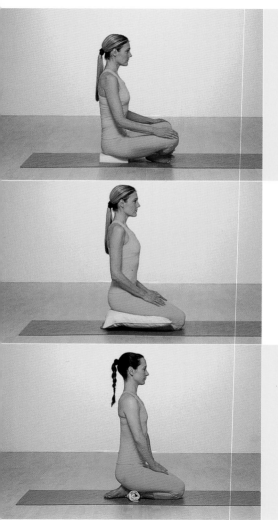

FOAM BLOCK

A firm foam block will help if your hips are stiff or you find it difficult to lengthen the spine in sitting postures, because it optimizes the tilt of the pelvis. If your neck is uncomfortable when you are lying on your back, you may find it useful to have a block as a support under your head.

PILLOW

A pillow can be used instead of a block to sit on or to rest your head on. It can also be used as a support to help relieve muscular tension. When kneeling, a pillow can be placed under the bent knees to help relieve tension in the inner thigh muscles.

ROLLED TOWEL

Kneeling positions can put strain on stiff ankles. To relieve this, roll up a towel firmly and place it between the ankles and the floor. A folded towel can also be used under bony parts of the feet or ankles, especially if you are working on a hard floor.

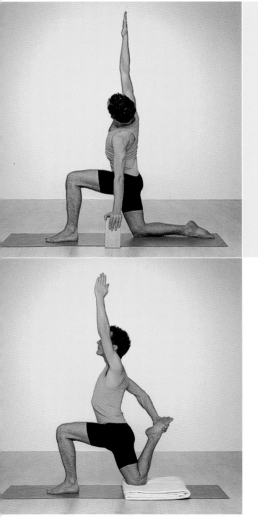

WOODEN BLOCK

Blocks can be used in a wide variety of situations as supports and stabilizers to help you practice postures effectively without straining yourself. If using a block in the Chandra sequence (see left and p.447) or Triangle (see p.402), consider the block as an extension of your arm, and position it carefully so that your final posture maintains alignment. Check the placing of the block before you move into your posture.

FOLDED BLANKET

A blanket can be used for support in sitting, kneeling, and inverted postures, and to keep warm in relaxation and meditation. In a state of deep relaxation, the body temperature can drop considerably, so it is wise to cover up with a blanket before you start practicing your relaxation technique.

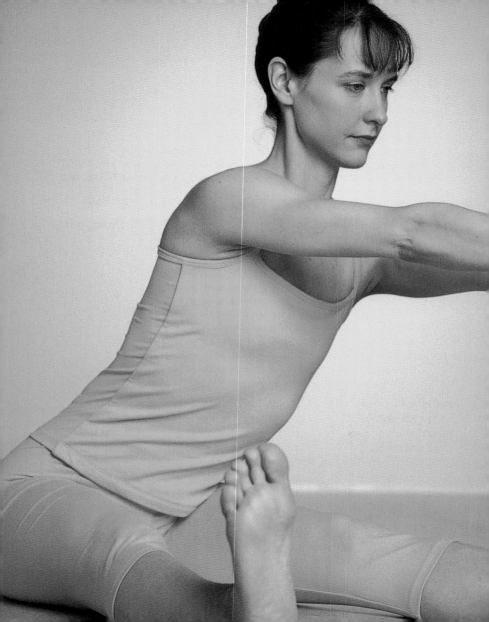

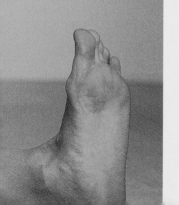

foundations

This section provides advice for those new to yoga. It includes some basic breathing techniques. It also contains breath-with-movement stretching exercises to loosen the body and help you deepen the connection with the breath.

basic
breathing

There is a fundamental connection between the breath and your physical, mental, and emotional states. In yoga, the breath is how vital energy – "the breath behind the breath" – enters the body.

Breathing well is of fundamental importance for health. Breathing provides oxygen for the metabolic processes from which we derive the energy to move, think, and feel and carries away carbon dioxide, the main waste product of metabolism. Physical tension in the respiratory muscles between the ribs can cause tightness in the chest, and even chest pain. Relaxed breathing techniques will release tension from the whole of the upper body, improving your ability to adjust your breathing to meet changing requirements.

The breath also provides a powerful link between mind and body. By controlling your breathing patterns – for example, the rhythm and depth of breathing, the length of the out-breath, and the balance between right and left nostrils – you can influence your physical, mental, and emotional states.

Good breathing habits

Yoga encourages breathing through the nose, full use of the diaphragm, a slow, smooth breathing pattern, and coordination of movement and breath. Opening movements, such as back bends, are practised on the in-breath, and closing movements, such as forward bends, on the out-breath.

Full Yogic Breath (see opposite) helps develop awareness of the action of respiratory muscles and encourages good breathing habits. It is essential to building self-esteem, and can be done lying down, standing, or sitting.

full yogic breath

This breathing practice induces calm, harmonizing breath and body. After completing Step 3, combine all three steps to produce full, continuous in- and out-breaths. This is called the complete breath. Do five rounds.

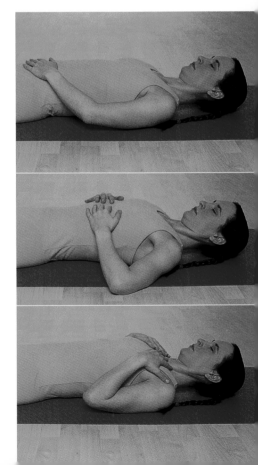

1 Lie on your back with your palms resting on your abdomen, the middle fingers just touching. Breathe into your hands, feeling the abdomen swell out and the fingers move apart as you breathe in. Then feel the abdomen sink back as you exhale. Repeat three times. This is abdominal breathing.

2 Bring your hands to your ribcage, with your fingers to the front and thumbs on the back ribs. On the in-breath, feel the ribs expand into the hands as the chest swells out. As you exhale, let the chest deflate and the hands sink down. Repeat three times like this.

3 Place your fingers on your collarbones, in front of your shoulders. Breathe in, and feel the the top of the chest expand and the fingers rise up toward the head. As you breathe out, feel the chest and fingers sink back down. Repeat three times like this.

breath with movement

These simple postures are designed to deepen your connection with your breath, as well as gently move your joints. Each movement is timed to match the length of the breath.

arm stretch 1

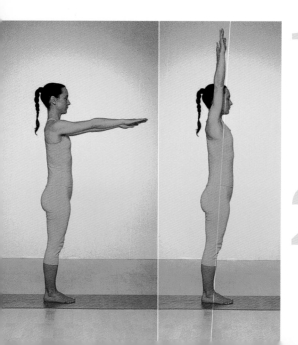

1 Practise the complete breath (see p.387) five times. Then, on an inhalation, raise the arms in front of you to shoulder height. Have the wrists, elbows, and shoulders in line, and the arms shoulder-width apart. Exhale.

2 On the next inhalation, extend the arms up directly above the head. Imagine a vertical line from your fingers to your ankles, aligning wrists, ears, and shoulders. Exhaling, return the arms to horizontal. Repeat the movement five times.

arm stretch 2

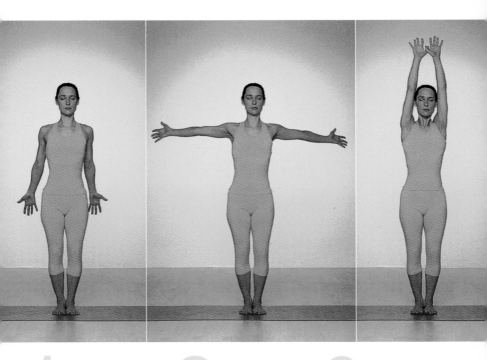

1 Stand with your feet together. As you exhale, turn the palms to face the front and pull the arms back, drawing the shoulder blades toward each other behind. Take a complete breath.

2 Starting to inhale, raise the arms up to shoulder height and out to the sides, extending the stretch right up to the fingertips. Keep the palms of the hands facing forward.

3 Still inhaling, extend the arms above your head, keeping them behind your ears. Feel the chest open. Exhale, lowering the arms by the sides, palms facing the front. Repeat the movement five times.

arm stretch 3

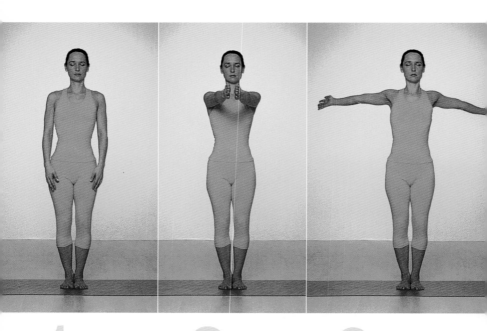

1 Stand up straight, feet together. Close your eyes. On an out-breath, release the shoulders down away from the ears. Let the palms rest on the thighs. Take a complete breath (see p.387), feeling it move through the body.

2 On an inhalation, let the arms float up to shoulder height. Turn the hands so the palms are facing each other and bring them close enough together to be able to feel the heat from each palm without the hands touching. Exhale.

3 As you inhale, open the arms out wide to the sides. Keep moving the arms back until you complete your inhalation with a fully open chest. Return to Step 2 as you exhale. Repeat Steps 2 and 3 seven times with your eyes closed.

energy-releasing pose

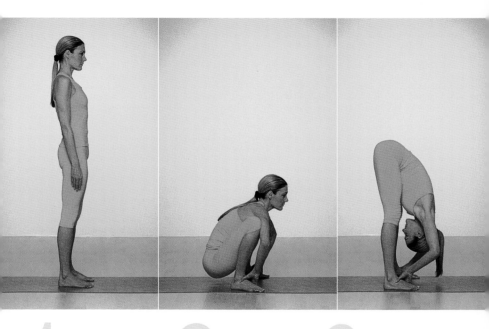

This practice develops synchronization between breath and movement, releasing energy and building strength. Stand with your feet hip-width apart, toes pointing forward, arms by your side. Look straight ahead and breathe in.

As you exhale, bend your knees and squat, tucking your fingers under the instep of each foot. Inhale, lengthening the spine and neck to look up. Point the elbows out and keep the tops of your thighs close to the lower belly.

As you exhale, straighten your legs, lifting your bottom toward the ceiling. Let your head hang down low so you can look between your calves. Keep the hands under the feet. Repeat Steps 2 and 3 five to seven times.

elbow circling

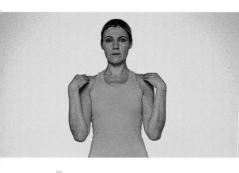 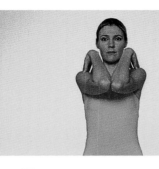

1 Breathing in, stretch out the arms in front of you. Turn the palms up, bend the elbows, and rest the fingers on the shoulders. Breathing out, let the elbows drop down to the waist.

2 On the next in-breath, lift the elbows out in front of your body at shoulder height, keeping the fingers on the shoulders. Pull the elbows toward each other until they touch.

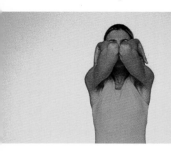 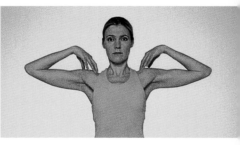

3 Still breathing in, lift the elbows higher in front of you, pointing them up toward the ceiling. Make sure the elbows do not separate.

4 As you breathe out, let the elbows separate and move the arms out at shoulder height. Roll the elbows back and down in a circular motion. Repeat Steps 2 to 4 three to seven times.

yogic rock and roll

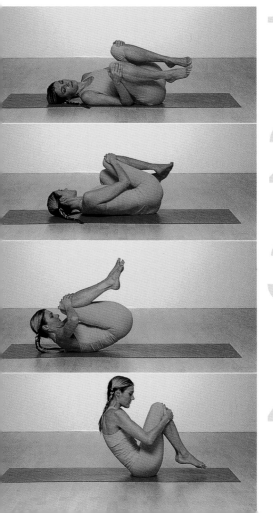

1 Lie on your back and take a complete breath (see p.387). On an in-breath, bend the knees and bring them up on each side of the abdomen. Hold a knee with each hand and rock to one side.

2 Breathing out, roll your body over to the other side. Roll from side to side like this several times. Then center your body.

3 As you breathe in, rock back gently along the length of the spine. Keep your back rounded and your legs tucked on each side of your abdomen.

4 As you breathe out, rock forward along the length of the spine. Rock back and forth like this several times. Finally, on an out-breath, come up to sitting.

pulling the rope

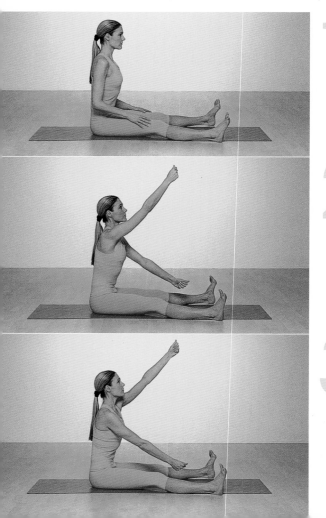

1 Sit with the legs straight out in front a little over hip-width apart. Keep the spine straight and lift up from the hips. Place your hands just above your knees. Flex your feet. Look straight ahead.

2 On an inhalation, reach your right hand up as high as it will go, and a little in front, as if to grab hold of an imaginary bell rope. Keep the arm straight and look up at the hand. Straighten and lift the left arm as if to hold the rope lower down.

3 On an exhalation, move the right hand down as if pulling the rope. Keep a stretch right through to the hand and move the trunk forward from the hips. Repeat Steps 2 and 3 on the left side. Then alternate right and left five to seven times.

rowing the boat

1 Sit with legs together, straight out in front. Push the heels away and lift up from the hips. Take an abdominal breath. Hold the arms out in front at shoulder level and make two fists as if holding the handles of a pair of oars. Exhale.

2 On an inhalation, lean back as far as you find comfortable, pulling the imaginary pair of oars. Bend the elbows and tuck them down into the waist. Feel the stretch in the abdomen.

3 On an exhalation, move the body forward as far as you can, reaching the arms straight out over the toes. Feel the stretch in the lower back. Repeat Steps 2 and 3 five to seven times, moving with the breath.

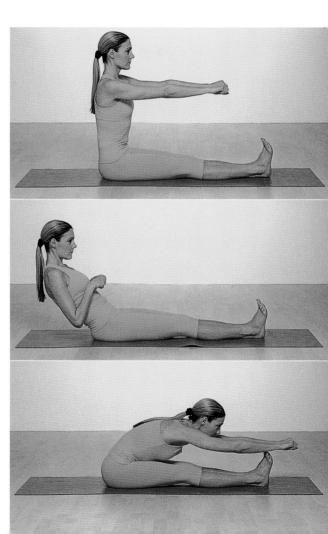

stirring the pot

1 Sit up straight, your legs in front as far apart as is comfortable. Sit forward on your sitting bones and extend your arms straight out in front, at shoulder height. Interlock your fingers so the right thumb is on top.

2 Imagine that you are holding a huge wooden spoon and that there is an enormous pot of oatmeal placed between your heels. Exhale as you move forward from the hips, keeping your arms at shoulder height.

3 Still exhaling, move your body and arms over your right foot. This is the beginning of a circular motion as you stir the imaginary pot of oatmeal between your heels.

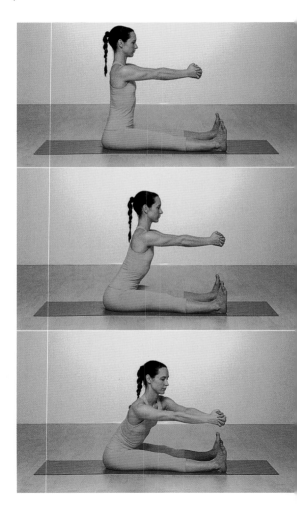

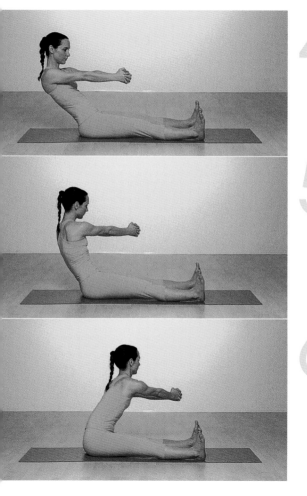

Continue in a clockwise direction. Inhale as you lean back, still moving from the hips, until your hands are positioned over your right thigh.

Still leaning back and breathing in, move your body to the left, bringing your hands over your left thigh. Feel the stretch in the pelvis and abdomen.

Breathing out, move your body forward so your hands are over your left foot. This completes one circle. Repeat the circular motion 10 times clockwise. Pause, resting your arms, and repeat 10 times, with the left thumb on top, in a counter-clockwise direction.

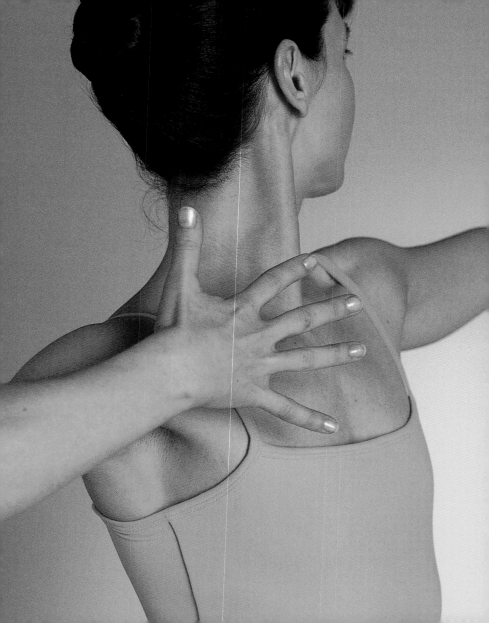

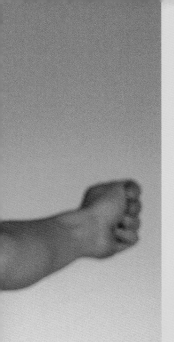

building blocks

This section presents a variety of postures and other yoga practices to promote awareness and develop self-confidence. Stay in the postures only for as long as you are able to hold them steadily and comfortably, breathing evenly. Listen to your body as you practice.

bow and
arrow

Promoting balanced strength, clear focus, and an open heart, this posture works deep into the muscles around the neck and shoulder blades to release tension and relieve stiffness and cramp.

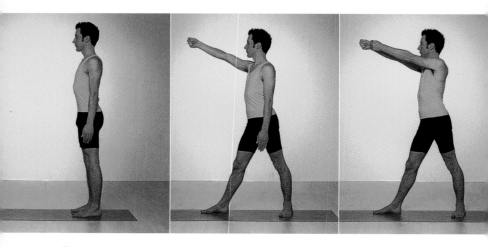

1 Stand with your feet shoulder-width apart, arms by your sides. Step the right foot forward 2 ft (60 cm). Turn the left foot out 45 degrees.

2 Clench your right hand and, inhaling, raise your right arm up and out above shoulder level, over the right foot. Gaze at the right thumb.

3 Tuck the thumb of the left hand into the palm and wrap the fingers around it. Exhaling, raise the left arm to bring the left hand up against the inside of the right wrist.

On the next inhalation, slowly bend the left elbow as you draw the left hand back to your chin and then behind the left ear, as though drawing on a bow. Tense the muscles in both arms. Exhale, and then take a breath in.

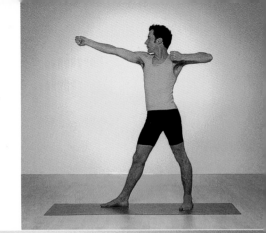

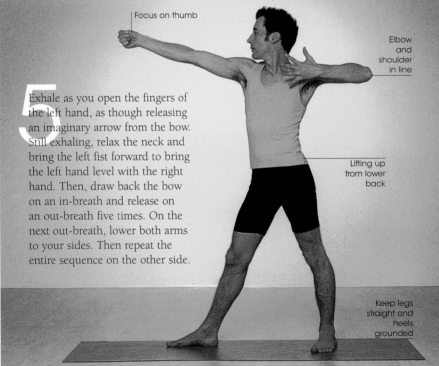

Focus on thumb

Elbow and shoulder in line

Exhale as you open the fingers of the left hand, as though releasing an imaginary arrow from the bow. Still exhaling, relax the neck and bring the left fist forward to bring the left hand level with the right hand. Then, draw back the bow on an in-breath and release on an out-breath five times. On the next out-breath, lower both arms to your sides. Then repeat the entire sequence on the other side.

Lifting up from lower back

Keep legs straight and heels grounded

triangle

Triangle builds physical strength, lifts the spirits, improves emotional confidence, and promotes balance. It stretches spine and abdomen, strengthens legs and feet, and promotes flexibility in the hips.

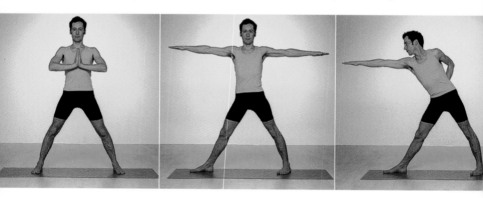

1 Stand with your feet about 3 ft (1 m) apart and bring your palms together in front of your chest. Exhale.

2 As you breathe in sweep your arms out to the side at shoulder height. Turn your right foot so the toes point to the side. Turn your left heel out.

3 As you exhale, reach out with the right arm, extending it as far as it will go. Bend the left arm and rest the palm of the hand in the small of the back.

TAKE CARE
• If you have back problems, rest front arm higher up the leg.
• Do not turn your head to look up at your hand if you have neck problems.

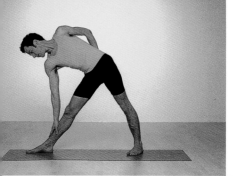

Still breathing out, lower the right arm to rest on the thigh and then slide it down the right leg. Keep the weight on the outside edges of your feet. Look at your right foot.

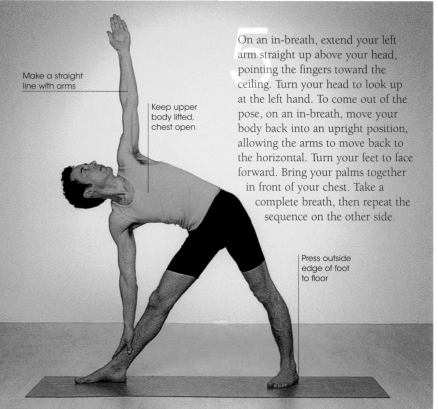

On an in-breath, extend your left arm straight up above your head, pointing the fingers toward the ceiling. Turn your head to look up at the left hand. To come out of the pose, on an in-breath, move your body back into an upright position, allowing the arms to move back to the horizontal. Turn your feet to face forward. Bring your palms together in front of your chest. Take a complete breath, then repeat the sequence on the other side.

Make a straight line with arms

Keep upper body lifted, chest open

Press outside edge of foot to floor

tree

An elegant balance, this posture promotes concentration and develops strength in the legs and feet. Coordinating the quietening of mind and body, Tree pose is an effective antidote to anxiety.

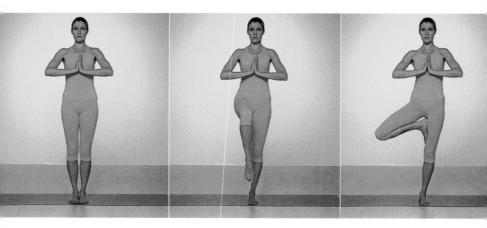

1 Stand with your legs and feet together. Bring your arms in front of your chest and push the heels of your hands firmly together, thumbs against chest. Inhale.

2 Exhale as you sink your weight into the left foot. On the next in-breath, raise the right knee up in front of you as high as it will comfortably go.

3 Turn the right knee out to the right side, and bring the sole of the right foot onto the inside of the left thigh. Keep your palms together. Take a complete breath.

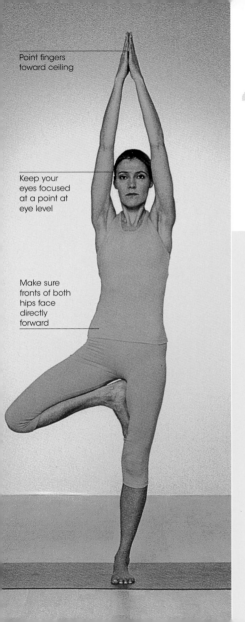

Point fingers toward ceiling

Keep your eyes focused at a point at eye level

Make sure fronts of both hips face directly forward

If you feel balanced, on the next inhalation, raise the hands up above the head, keeping the palms together and holding your focus on a point straight ahead. Take a complete breath. To come out of the pose, on an exhalation, bring the arms back down to your sides and lower your right foot to the floor. Take a few rounds of breath, then repeat the pose on the other side.

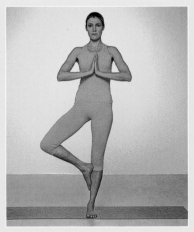

ALTERNATIVE

If you find it difficult to balance in the full pose, try bringing the sole of your right foot to rest just below the knee. If you have HBP, do not raise your arms above your head. Avoid the pose if you have arthritis in the knees or back problems.

dancer

This strong and energizing practice opens the chest and promotes excellent coordination and balance. The pose of the Dancer develops focus together with strength of mind and body.

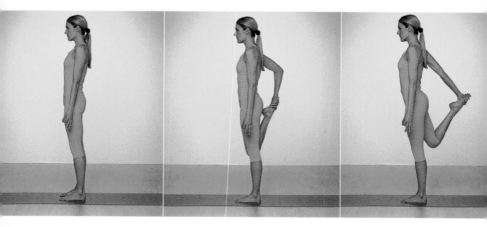

Stand with your legs together, arms by your sides. Look straight ahead. Press the tip of the left thumb against the tip of the left index finger, to make a circle. Exhale.

Bend the right knee and take the right foot behind you, catching hold of it with your right hand. Hold the foot close to the right buttock. Take a breath in.

On the next out-breath, slowly raise the right knee behind you to a comfortable height, still holding the foot. Keep your balance steady and your eyes focused.

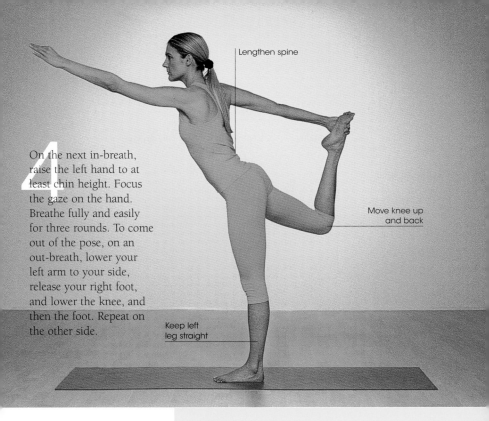

Lengthen spine

4 On the next in-breath, raise the left hand to at least chin height. Focus the gaze on the hand. Breathe fully and easily for three rounds. To come out of the pose, on an out-breath, lower your left arm to your side, release your right foot, and lower the knee, and then the foot. Repeat on the other side.

Move knee up and back

Keep left leg straight

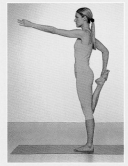

TAKE CARE
• Be careful not to collapse the back in the full pose: keep the back lengthened.
• Raise the knee behind you only as high as is comfortable.

ALTERNATIVE
If you find it difficult to raise the knee behind you in the full pose without losing balance, practice with the knees side-by-side. Work slowly to bring the heel close to the buttock, feeling the stretch in the thigh.

boat

An instant energizer that builds strength, promotes confidence, and develops concentration, Boat pose strengthens abdominal, back, and leg muscles, boosts circulation, and helps eliminate anxiety.

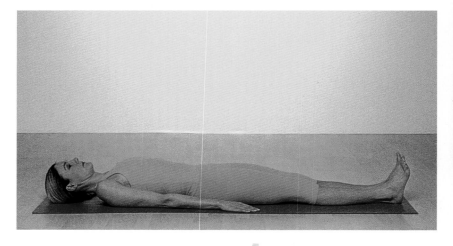

TAKE CARE
Avoid this practice if you have HBP, a heart condition, slipped disk, or sciatica.

1 Lie on your back, with your arms by your sides, shoulders well away from your ears, and palms down. Have your legs straight and together. Observe the rise and fall of the abdominal breath (see p.387).

Keeping your focus on the abdomen, take a deep breath in and hold it inside as you raise your arms, shoulders, head, trunk, and legs up about 4 in (10 cm) off the ground. Keeping your arms and legs straight, extend your hands toward the toes and draw the toes in toward your head. Keep the hands and feet at roughly the same height as you balance on your buttocks.

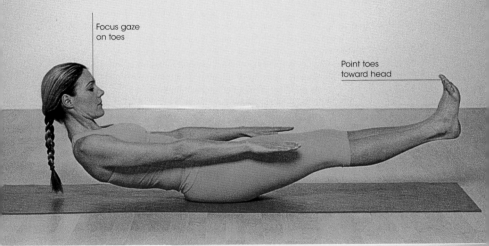

Focus gaze on toes

Point toes toward head

When you are ready to exhale, slowly lower the legs, trunk, and head back onto the floor. Rest with arms and legs by your sides to release all body tension. Repeat three to five times.

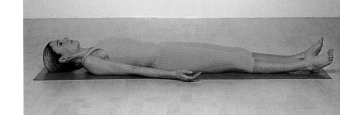

downward
dog

An invigorating stretch, Downward Dog strengthens the limbs and relieves tightness in the back and shoulders. This classic inversion is a powerful energy booster.

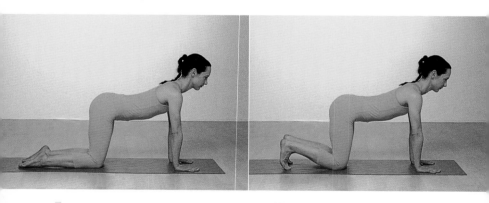

1 Begin on all fours, the hands directly under the shoulders, the feet and knees hip-width apart. Look slightly ahead. Take a breath in.

2 Maintaining the position of your hands and knees, lift your feet and tuck your toes under. Continue to look at the floor slightly ahead.

TAKE CARE
• If you have a back problem, do the posture cautiously with your knees bent throughout.
• If you have HBP, a heart condition, glaucoma, or a detached retina, do the posture with your hands on a chair.

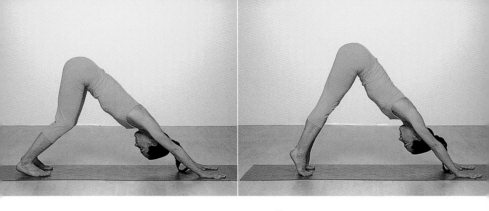

3 On an out-breath, lift your hips up and back. Keeping your knees bent, push your hands against the floor to send your weight back toward your feet. Lengthen through the spine. Let your head hang between your arms.

4 Straighten your legs, coming up onto your toes as you lift your sitting bones up toward the ceiling. Lengthen through your back and keep your neck relaxed and your head hanging. Take a breath in.

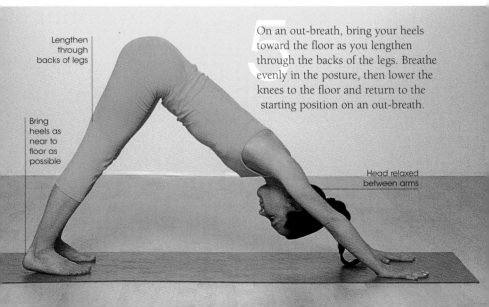

Lengthen through backs of legs

Bring heels as near to floor as possible

5 On an out-breath, bring your heels toward the floor as you lengthen through the backs of the legs. Breathe evenly in the posture, then lower the knees to the floor and return to the starting position on an out-breath.

Head relaxed between arms

lunge
warrior

A powerful and poised practice, Lunge Warrior promotes flexibility in the hips and opens the hips and thighs. It also encourages steady focus and stability of balance.

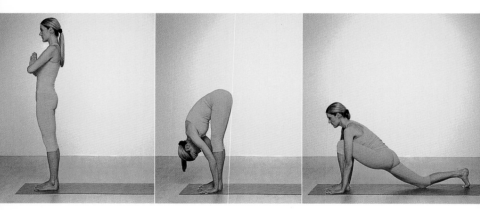

1 Stand up straight, feet together, arms by your side. Bring your palms together in front of your chest.

2 As you breathe out, fold your body forward from the hips, bending the knees slightly. Place your palms on the floor on each side of your feet. Take a breath in.

3 As you breathe out, bend the knees, and take a large step back with your right foot. Land on the ball of the right foot. Rest your upper body on your left thigh. Look slightly ahead.

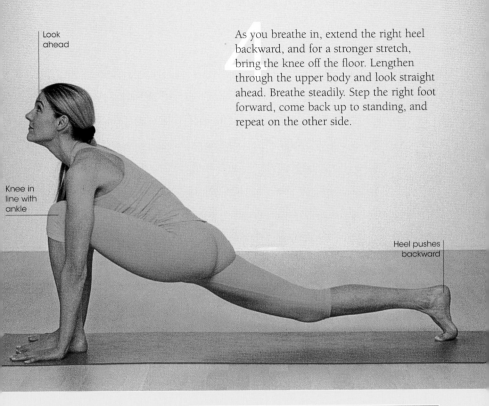

Look
ahead

Knee in
line with
ankle

Heel pushes
backward

As you breathe in, extend the right heel
backward, and for a stronger stretch,
bring the knee off the floor. Lengthen
through the upper body and look straight
ahead. Breathe steadily. Step the right foot
forward, come back up to standing, and
repeat on the other side.

ALTERNATIVE

If you have back problems,
HBP, or a heart condition, do
not lift your right knee off the
ground in the full pose. Allow
the weight of the hips to sink
down and through into the
grounded knee.

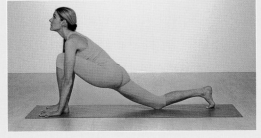

cobra

Cobra extends the spine, strengthening the back muscles and opening the chest. It is a valuable posture for developing a sense of power and grace, boosting self-confidence.

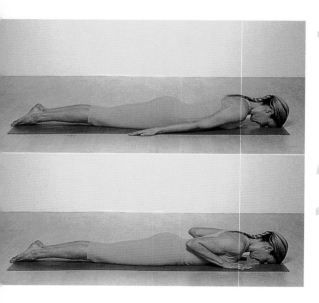

1 Lie on your front, forehead on the floor and feet together with heels touching. Let your arms lie down by your sides, palms facing down. Exhale.

2 Place your hands under the shoulders, spread your fingers, middle finger pointing forward. Keep the elbows close to the body and tuck your tailbone under.

TAKE CARE
• Avoid if you have facet joint problems in the spine.
• If you have arthritis in the neck, keep the head in line with the spine.

As you breathe in, slide the forehead forward to lift the forehead, nose, chin, and then the shoulders and chest. Use the back muscles to lift the upper body off the floor. Focus on taking the chest forward, lengthening through the front of the body and extending throughout the spine. Breathe easily. There should be no feeling of strain.

Extend
spine

Relax
shoulders

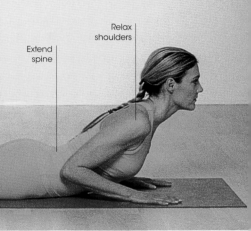

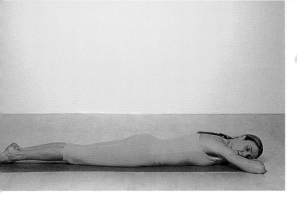

Repeat the pose once or twice, then relax for a few minutes. Bring your arms forward, and fold one under the other. Turn your head to one side and rest your face on your forearms. Close your eyes.

snake

This backward bend stretches the front of the body, opens the chest, and promotes easeful movement in the upper back. Taking the arms back helps relieve stiffness in the shoulders and the mid-back.

1 Lie flat on your front with your forehead on the floor and your arms by your sides, palms facing down. Have your legs straight, your heels together. Exhale.

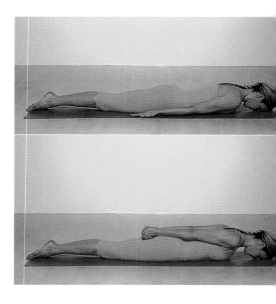

2 Breathing in, lift your arms up and bring them behind your back. Move your elbows as close together as you can. Place the palms of your hands together and interlock the fingers. Roll your shoulders down and back away from your ears, squeezing your shoulder blades together. Exhale.

TAKE CARE
Do not practice this posture if you have a peptic ulcer or a hernia.

3 As you breathe in, lift your head and raise the front of your chest up away from the floor. Look straight ahead. Exhale.

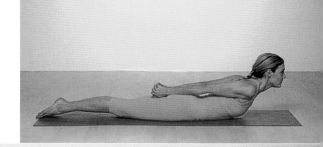

4 On the next inhalation, lift the arms up away from the back and move your hands away toward your feet. Keep the arms and hands together. Hold the posture for up to seven complete breaths. Feel your abdomen moving against the floor as you breathe.

Keep neck long and shoulders well away from ears

Squeeze shoulder blades together

Keep heels pressing together

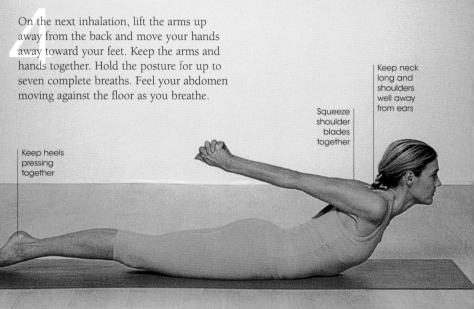

5 On an exhalation, slowly lower the arms down onto the back, tuck in the chin, and rest the forehead on the floor.

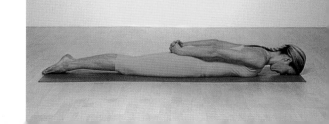

resting crocodile

Resting Crocodile is a healing posture for many types of back pain, including slipped disc, sciatica, and lower back pain. It also encourages full and complete breathing.

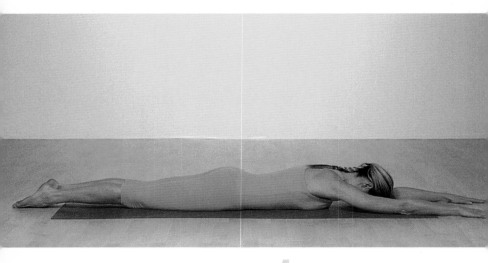

TAKE CARE
• Let your feet and ankles relax. Point toes in toward each other or out to the sides.
• Feel the abdomen moving against the floor as you inhale.

1 Lie flat on your front, your feet hip-width apart and your arms outstretched above your head. Rest your forehead on the floor. This is known as the Reverse Corpse pose.

2 On an in-breath, bend your elbows, and bring the heels of your hands together. Raise your head and shoulders, and rest your chin in the palms of your hands. Stay in the posture for several breaths.

Gaze straight ahead

Upper back at a comfortable angle

Legs and buttocks relaxed

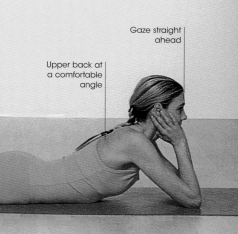

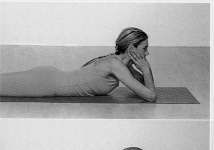

ALTERNATIVES

Take your elbows wider apart to spread the upper back and neck. Move your elbows further in front to lessen the angle of the curve in your back. Bring the elbows closer to the body to increase the angle of the curve in your back.

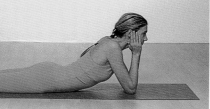

sun salute

The Sun Salute synchronizes breath with movement and promoting fluidity, endurance, strength, and adaptability. Best practiced early in the day, it harmonizes and energizes the whole body system.

1 Stand tall, with feet together and chest lifted. Inhale. On the out-breath, bring the palms of the hands together in the center of the chest in prayer position. Breathe into the heart space.

2 On the next in-breath, lift your hands over the head, straightening the arms, and turn the palms to face the sun in front of you. Lean back a little. Open the chest with your in-breath to feel strong and confident.

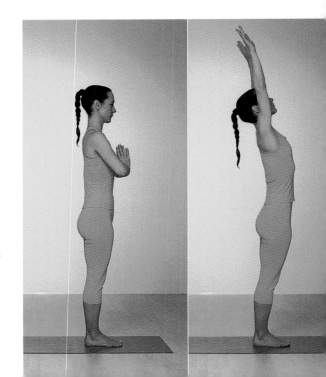

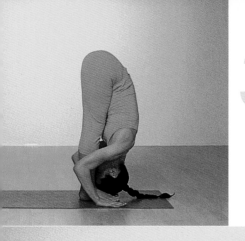

Exhaling, bend forward from the hips into a Forward Bend. Keep a long spine and bend your knees if you need to. Maintain a sense of one continuous line from the bottom of your spine to the tips of your fingers. Bring the hands flat on the floor on each side of your feet, fingers pointing forward. Tuck your head into your shins. Be soft.

On the next in-breath, keeping your palms flat on the floor, step your right leg as far back as you can into Lunge Warrior (see p.412). Let the right knee bend and rest on the floor. Keep the toes tucked under. If you need to, steeple the fingers. Bring your chest forward and draw your focus up to the point between your eyebrows as you raise your face up to soak up the energizing rays of the sun. ▶

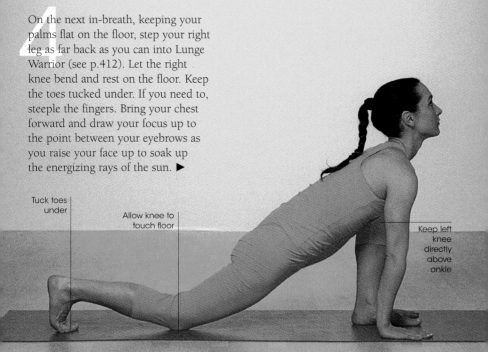

Tuck toes under

Allow knee to touch floor

Keep left knee directly above ankle

5 On the next exhalation, bring your left foot back to join your right, straighten your knees, and swing your tailbone up high. Straighten your arms and lift your shoulders back away from your ears. Lift up on your toes, and then lengthen through the backs of the legs to bring the heels down toward the floor into Downward Dog (see p.410).

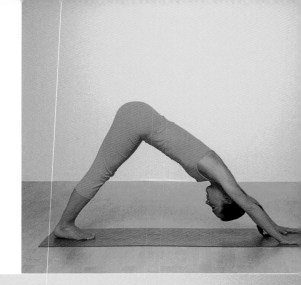

6 Let there be a pause in the breath as you lower your chest to the floor. Lower the head so that the nose touches the floor, too. Keep your bottom in the air and bend your knees until they touch the floor. Focus your attention on your abdomen.

Lift buttocks toward ceiling

Lower chest to floor directly between hands

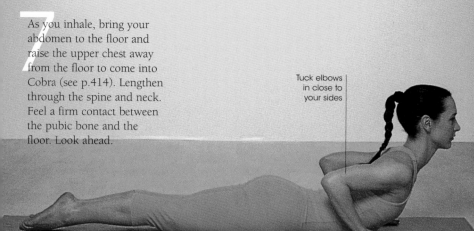

7 As you inhale, bring your abdomen to the floor and raise the upper chest away from the floor to come into Cobra (see p.414). Lengthen through the spine and neck. Feel a firm contact between the pubic bone and the floor. Look ahead.

Tuck elbows in close to your sides

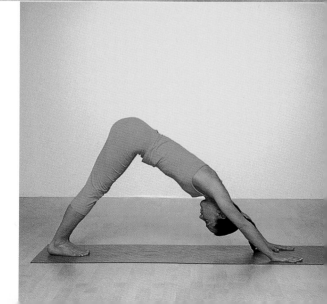

8 On the next exhalation, come into Downward Dog again. Tuck your toes under, straighten your knees, and swing your tailbone up high. Straighten your arms and move your shoulders back away from your ears. Lift up on your toes, and then lengthen through the backs of the legs to bring the heels down toward the floor. Let your head hang down between your arms. Relax the neck. ▶

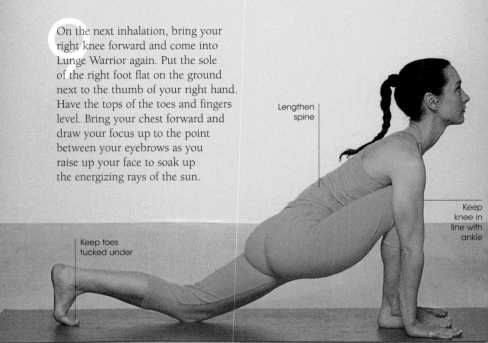

On the next inhalation, bring your right knee forward and come into Lunge Warrior again. Put the sole of the right foot flat on the ground next to the thumb of your right hand. Have the tops of the toes and fingers level. Bring your chest forward and draw your focus up to the point between your eyebrows as you raise up your face to soak up the energizing rays of the sun.

Lengthen spine

Keep knee in line with ankle

Keep toes tucked under

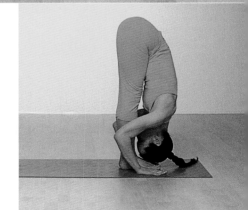

On the next exhalation, come back into a Forward Bend, bringing your left foot forward to join your right. Keep your hands flat on the floor, fingers pointing forward, and bend your knees if you need to. Have your head tucked into your shins and keep the focus of your attention at the base of your spine. Be soft, accepting of where you are able to be in the pose.

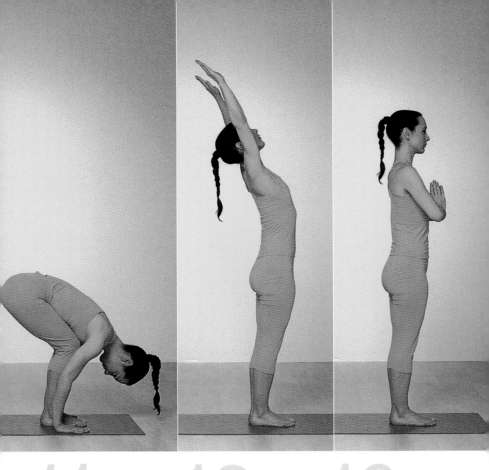

11 On the next in-breath, bend your knees and start to lift your body back up to standing, pivoting from the hips and keeping neck in line with spine.

12 Continuing to breathe in, bring your arms up above your head. Keeping the arms straight and long, lean back a little and open your chest to feel strong and confident.

13 On the next in-breath, bring the palms together above the head. Breathing out, lower them until they come to the center of the chest. Breathe into the heart space.

thunderbolt

This useful meditation posture aligns the spine, neck, and head, and promotes flexibility in the ankles and feet. The quiet that it brings to the body is conducive to digestion.

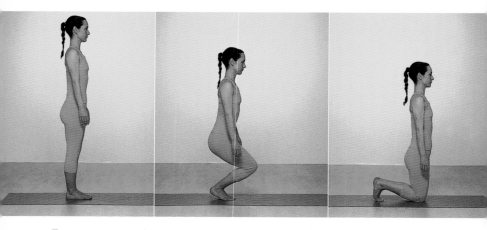

1 Stand with your feet together and arms by your sides. Look straight ahead. Inhale.

2 As you exhale, keeping your knees together, lower them forward and down to the floor.

3 With your thighs vertical, bring the big toes together and the heels apart. Untuck the toes so the tops of the feet are on the floor. Keep the spine straight. Inhale.

As you exhale, lower your buttocks onto the feet and let your heels touch the sides of your hips. Place your hands just above your knees, palms down. Breathe evenly for a few minutes. To come out of the posture, tuck the toes under and lift the knees up off the floor. On an inhalation, return to standing.

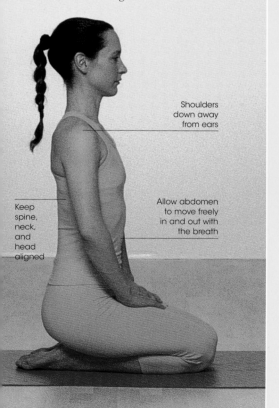

Shoulders down away from ears

Keep spine, neck, and head aligned

Allow abdomen to move freely in and out with the breath

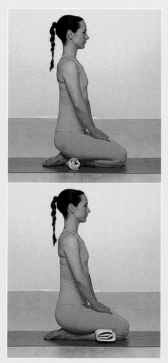

ALTERNATIVES

If you find that your ankles ache, tuck a rolled blanket in the front of the ankle joint, between ankle and floor. If you have varicose veins or knee problems, try tucking a rolled blanket between your knees and your calves. If you feel any discomfort in the thighs, separate the knees slightly.

philosopher

A rapid route to physical and mental relaxation, this pose develops the powers of concentration and enables clarity of thought. It encourages a quiet, contemplative self-confidence.

1 Start by kneeling in Thunderbolt pose (see p.426) with your knees together and the palms of your hands resting on your thighs. Sit back on your heels and straighten your spine. Look straight ahead. Take a complete breath. As you exhale, settle your weight down. Let your awareness travel within.

TAKE CARE
Keep the spine and neck extended, feeling a continuous line from the tailbone to the top of the head.

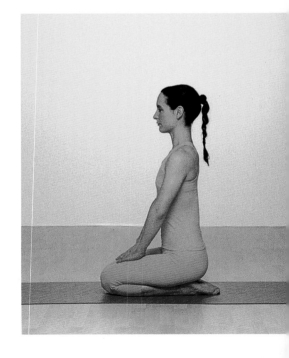

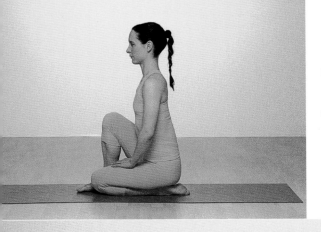

2 Inhale as you lift up the right knee, and put the sole of the right foot flat on the floor to the inside of the left knee, bringing the right ankle directly underneath the right knee.

3 Exhaling, raise your right elbow and place it on top of the right knee. Rest your chin on the palm of the right hand. Close your eyes and focus on your breathing for two minutes, imagining that the breath is flowing in and out through a point between your eyebrows. To come out of the pose, lower the right hand and your right knee, and repeat on the left side.

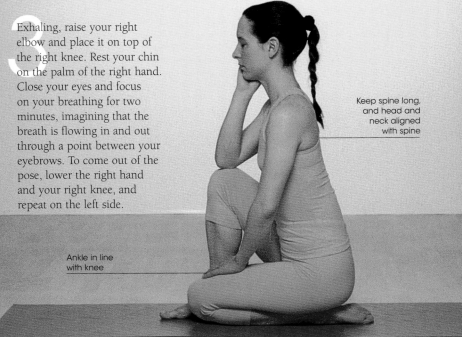

Keep spine long, and head and neck aligned with spine

Ankle in line with knee

roaring
lion

A potent antidote to introversion, this pose promotes a beautiful voice and gives you the confidence to use it. It stretches the face, jaw, and throat and releases tension in the chest.

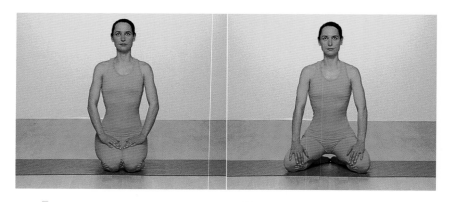

1 Kneel in Thunderbolt (see p.426) with your knees together and the palms of your hands on your thighs. If possible, face the sun. Inhale.

2 Exhale as you move your knees about 18 in (45 cm) apart. Spread out your fingers just above your knees, keeping your thumbs closest to your body.

TAKE CARE
• When you are comfortable with the practice, you may do up to 20 repetitions.
• If you have knee problems or painful wrists, sit on a chair. Lean forward, the hands placed lightly on the thighs.

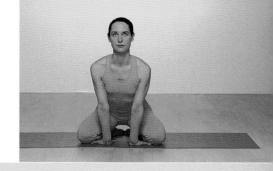

3 Place your palms flat on the floor in between your knees with your fingers pointing back toward your body. Inhale. Lower your shoulders and keep your spine long and straight as you lean forward slightly. Exhale.

4 Push the chest forward as you inhale deeply through the nose. At the end of the inhalation, open your mouth as wide as possible and stick out your tongue, stretching the tip down toward your chin. On the exhalation, emit a long, breathy "aaaahhh" sound, like a soft roar, from the back of your throat. Feel the sound and the breath pouring out along the tongue. At the end of the "aaaahhh," put your tongue back inside the mouth and close the lips. Repeat the roar between three and seven times.

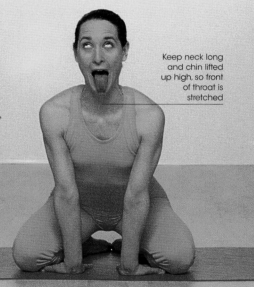

Keep neck long and chin lifted up high, so front of throat is stretched

5 When you have completed your chosen number of rounds, release the hands and, on an exhalation, fold forward from the hips to bring your forehead to the floor and arms beside your body. Stay for several breaths.

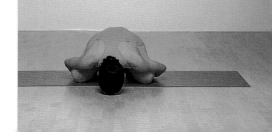

camel

Energizing and revitalizing, this powerful backward bend requires and promotes confidence and trust. It stretches the front of the body and opens the chest, relieving tension in the upper back.

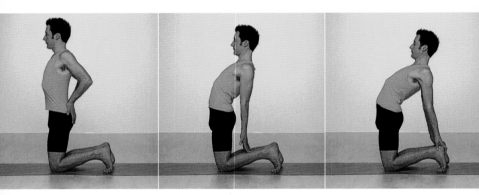

1 Kneel with knees hip-width apart. Tuck the toes under. Place your palms on the buttocks. Breathe in.

2 Keeping the spine extended, slowly move the hands down your thighs until they reach the shins.

3 Push the chest forward with an out-breath and grasp the heels. Draw the shoulder blades together behind you, opening the chest.

TAKE CARE
• If you have HBP, heart disease, back problems, hernia, or have had recent abdominal surgery, do not go beyond Step 2.
• If you have neck problems, do not take head back at Step 4.

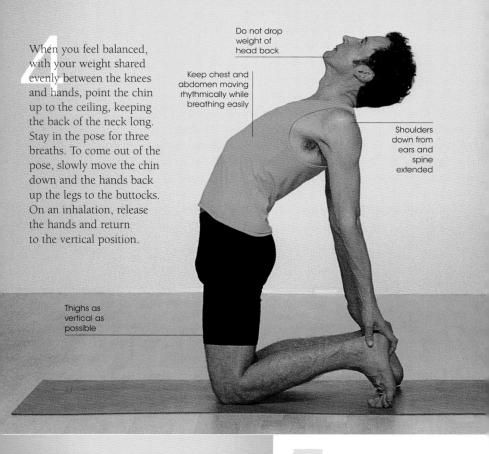

When you feel balanced, with your weight shared evenly between the knees and hands, point the chin up to the ceiling, keeping the back of the neck long. Stay in the pose for three breaths. To come out of the pose, slowly move the chin down and the hands back up the legs to the buttocks. On an inhalation, release the hands and return to the vertical position.

Do not drop weight of head back

Keep chest and abdomen moving rhythmically while breathing easily

Shoulders down from ears and spine extended

Thighs as vertical as possible

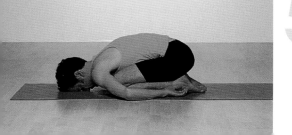

On an exhalation, fold forward into Child (see p.436) and lengthen the spine. Breathe into the abdomen and feel it moving against the thighs. Rest in this pose for a few minutes.

cat

Synchronizing breath and movement, Cat pose creates a strong link between mind and body. It eases tension in the spine and develops a full and effective yogic breath (see p.387).

1 Start in the all-fours position, with the palms flat on the floor directly under the shoulders and the fingers well spread and pointing forward. Push the hands into the floor to prevent the shoulders from sagging. Look down at the floor. Take an in-breath.

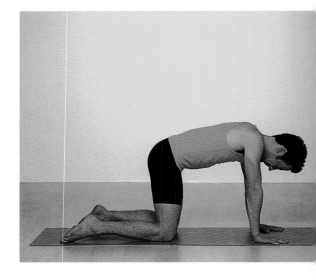

TAKE CARE
If you have weak wrists, support the body by placing one or both forearms on a pile of blocks or books.

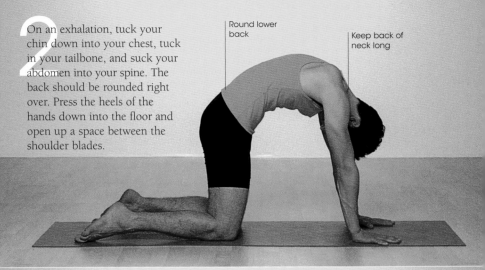

2 On an exhalation, tuck your chin down into your chest, tuck in your tailbone, and suck your abdomen into your spine. The back should be rounded right over. Press the heels of the hands down into the floor and open up a space between the shoulder blades.

Round lower back

Keep back of neck long

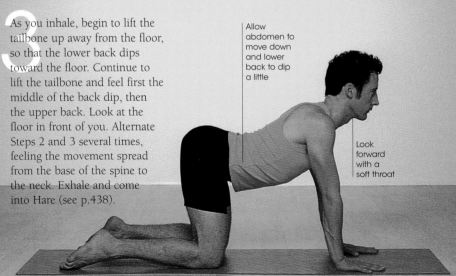

3 As you inhale, begin to lift the tailbone up away from the floor, so that the lower back dips toward the floor. Continue to lift the tailbone and feel first the middle of the back dip, then the upper back. Look at the floor in front of you. Alternate Steps 2 and 3 several times, feeling the movement spread from the base of the spine to the neck. Exhale and come into Hare (see p.438).

Allow abdomen to move down and lower back to dip a little

Look forward with a soft throat

child

Quietening and calming, Child pose provides a long stretch through the spine and easeful rest for shoulders and neck. It is excellent for developing awareness of the abdominal breath (see p.387).

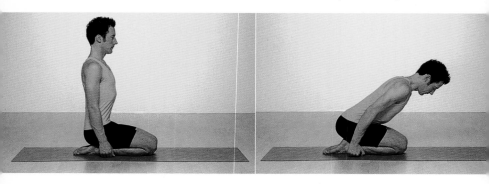

1 Kneel and sit back on your heels. Let your arms hang down on each side of the body. Lengthen through the spine and look straight ahead. Breathe in.

2 As you breathe out, fold forward slowly from the hips. Keep your buttocks on your heels and your arms by your sides.

TAKE CARE
• If you cannot sit on your heels, place a pillow beneath the buttocks.
• If you find it difficult to bring your head to the floor, rest it on two fists, one on top of the other. • If you have HBP, a detached retina, glaucoma, or back problems, rest your head on the seat of a chair.

Continue to fold forward, tucking the chin in to bring the forehead to the floor. Allow the weight of the arms to pull the shoulders gently toward the floor. Stay for several breaths.

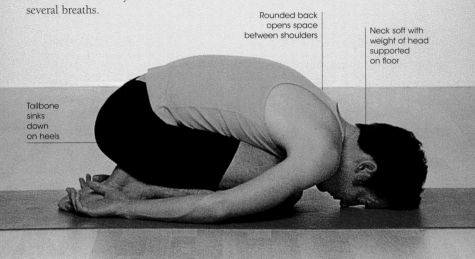

Rounded back opens space between shoulders

Neck soft with weight of head supported on floor

Tailbone sinks down on heels

To come out of the pose, on an in-breath, bring the palms of your hands to the floor and begin to push up slowly. Gradually come back up to kneeling, your arms by your side, back straight.

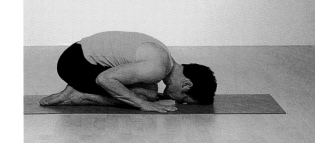

hare

This peaceful pose is soothing and quietening, providing relief from harsh self-criticism and anger. It also stretches the back and helps encourage good alignment of the spine.

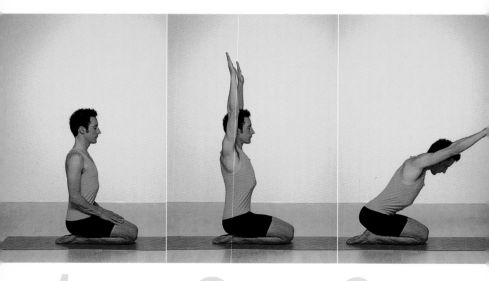

1 Sit in Thunderbolt pose (see p.426). Keep your back long and rest the palms of your hands on the thighs.

2 Inhale as you raise your arms above the head. Make a straight line from fingertips to the base of the spine.

3 Exhale as you fold forward from the hips, extending the fingertips forward as you come down.

4 Bring your forehead and the palms of your hands to rest on the floor at the same time. Extend the arms away in front of you, feeling an open space under your armpits. Breathe fully and easily in the pose. On an inhalation, keeping the head between the arms, and the back straight, return to a vertical position.

Allow upper back to open and relax

Extend arms forward

Sink weight of buttocks down onto heels

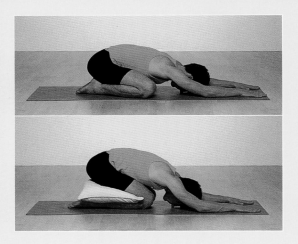

ALTERNATIVES

If you find it uncomfortable to keep your knees together, allow them to come a little apart. If you are not comfortable sitting back on your heels, place a pillow between your heels and your buttocks. If you have HBP, a detached retina, glaucoma, or back problems, stretch forward with your hands on the seat of a chair.

chandra
sequence

Requiring and promoting balance and strength, this sequence encourages fluidity of movement and sustained self-awareness. It energizes and releases the pelvic area.

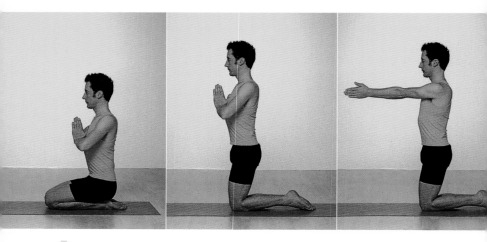

1 Start in Thunderbolt (see p.426). Bring the arms in front of your chest and press the heels of the hands together in prayer position. Exhale.

2 Inhale as you rise up onto the knees, keeping your back straight and your hands in front of you in prayer position.

3 As you breathe out, straighten your arms out in front of you, palms still pressed together, fingers pointing away from the body.

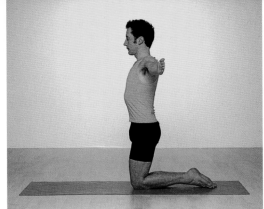

As you inhale, open your arms wide to the sides at shoulder height, keeping your arms straight.

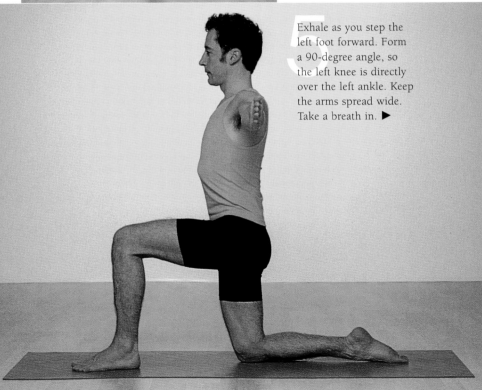

Exhale as you step the left foot forward. Form a 90-degree angle, so the left knee is directly over the left ankle. Keep the arms spread wide. Take a breath in. ▶

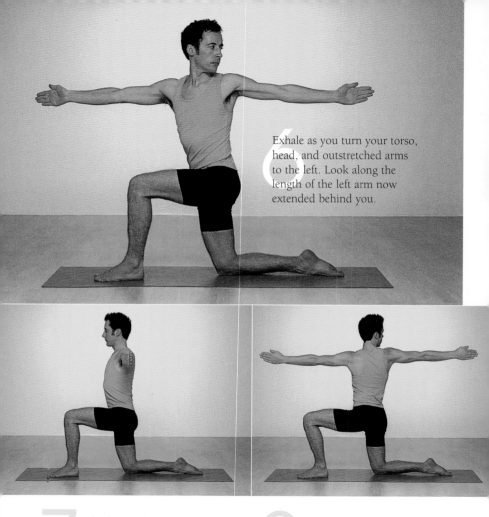

Exhale as you turn your torso, head, and outstretched arms to the left. Look along the length of the left arm now extended behind you.

Keeping both arms held out straight and at shoulder height, breathe in as you return to the front. Look directly in front of you.

Exhale as you turn your torso, head, and outstretched arms to the right. Look along the length of the right arm. Keep both arms straight and at shoulder height.

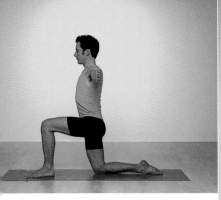

9 Keeping both arms straight and at shoulder height, inhale as you return to the front. Look directly in front of you.

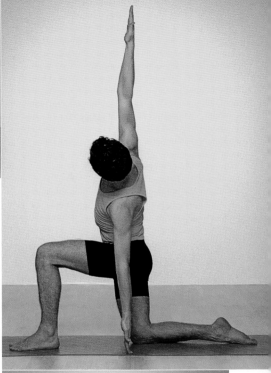

10 Exhale as you bend at the waist to bring the left arm down to touch the floor with your fingertips. Stretch the right arm up, keeping a long straight line from the right fingertips to the left. Look up at the right hand. Take a breath in as you return to the centre, keeping the arms wide.

11 Exhale as you bend at the waist to bring the right arm down to touch the floor with your fingertips. Stretch the left arm up, keeping a straight line from the left fingertips to the right. Look up at the left hand. Come back to Step 9 on the in-breath. ▶

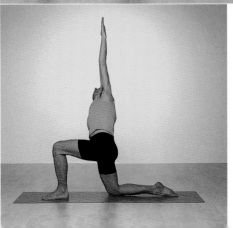

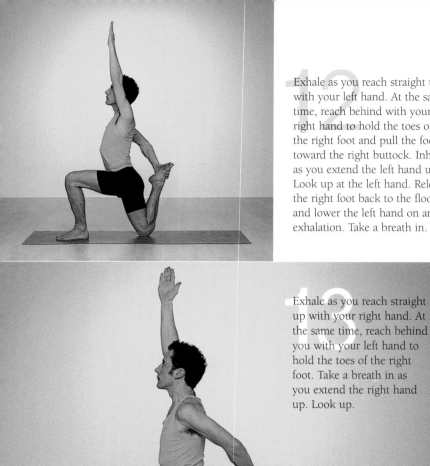

Exhale as you reach straight up with your left hand. At the same time, reach behind with your right hand to hold the toes of the right foot and pull the foot up toward the right buttock. Inhale as you extend the left hand up. Look up at the left hand. Release the right foot back to the floor and lower the left hand on an exhalation. Take a breath in.

Exhale as you reach straight up with your right hand. At the same time, reach behind you with your left hand to hold the toes of the right foot. Take a breath in as you extend the right hand up. Look up.

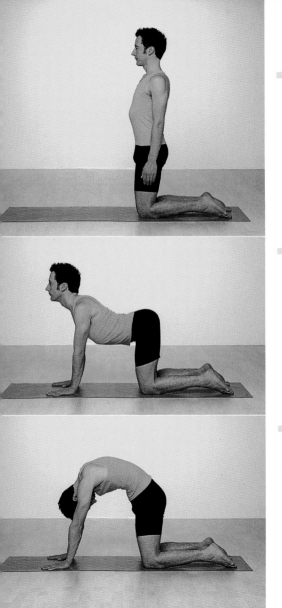

Release the right foot back to the floor and lower the right hand on an exhalation. Inhale. Exhale as you step your left foot back to return to Thunderbolt pose.

Bend at the waist to come down onto all fours. Have the palms flat on the floor directly under the shoulders, with the fingers spread and pointing forward. Inhale fully as you look forward and slightly up, lengthening through the whole spine as it dips slightly in Step 3 of Cat (see p.435).

On an exhalation, tuck your chin down into your chest, tuck in your tailbone, and suck your abdomen up to your spine in Step 2 of Cat. Press the heels of the hands down into the floor and open up a space between your shoulder blades. Inhale and look forward to come back to Step 15. ▶

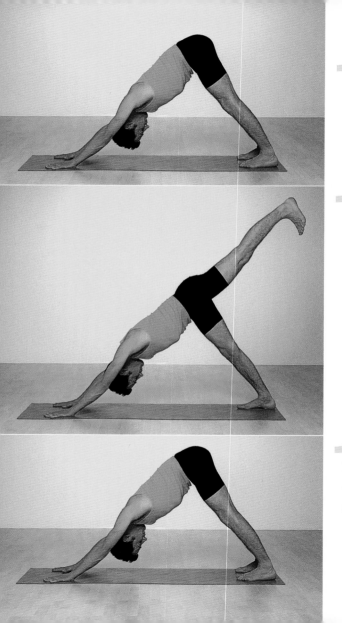

17 Exhale as you tuck your toes under and swing your tailbone up into Downward Dog (see p.410). Keep the elbows and knees strong and arms and legs straight.

18 Inhale as you raise the left leg up behind you, flexing the foot. Keep your neck relaxed and let your head hang between your arms.

19 Exhale as you place your left foot back on the floor, returning to Downward Dog. Take a full breath.

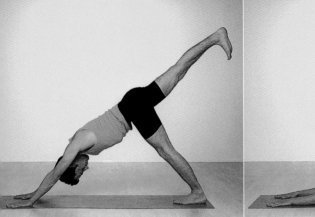

Inhale as you raise the right leg up behind you, flexing the foot. Exhale as you place your foot back on the floor. Breathe in.

Exhale as you bend your knees and lower your head to the floor, coming into Hare (see p.438). On an in-breath, come back up into Thunderbolt and repeat the sequence on the other side.

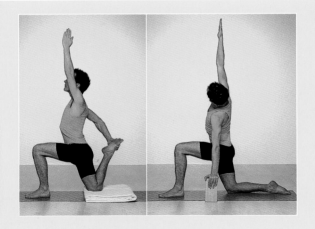

ALTERNATIVES

• If your knee feels uncomfortable in Steps 12 and 13, place a folded blanket beneath it. Have the blanket in place at the start of the sequence.

• If it is difficult to touch the floor in Steps 10 and 11 without losing balance, position a wooden block so you can rest the heel of your hand on it.

dolphin

The Dolphin pose is a vital part of the preparation for Headstand (see p.450). Until you can comfortably do 10 repetitions of this posture, you should not attempt to do Headstand.

1 Kneel on the floor with your hands resting lightly on your thighs and your buttocks resting on your heels. Inhale and then fold forward on an out-breath.

2 Inhale as you come on to your knees and elbows. Place your elbows under your shoulders and clasp each elbow with a hand.

3 Keeping the elbows still, slide your hands forward and interlock your fingers. Lift your shoulders back and down.

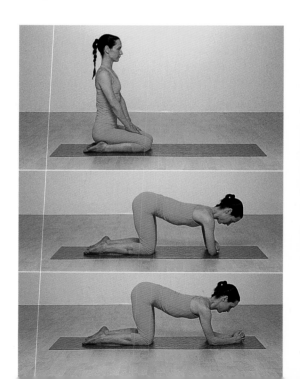

Breathing in, tuck your toes under and straighten your legs, so your buttocks lift and you feel the weight resting on your elbows and forearms. Keep your fingers interlocked.

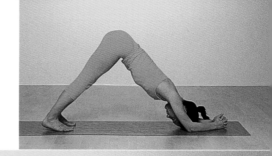

Raise your head. As you breathe in, move your head and shoulders forward until the shoulders are over the hands. Feel the weight descending into your elbows and forearms. As you exhale, move back. If you can, repeat the move: inhale forward and exhale back. To come out of the pose, move back onto all fours, then bring your buttocks back onto the heels and rest in Hare (see p.438).

Keep head and neck parallel to floor as you move forward and backward

Keep shoulders down away from ears

TAKE CARE
• Avoid Dolphin if you have HBP, heart disease, glaucoma, or a detached retina.
• Avoid the pose if you are menstruating.

headstand

This is the "king" of all yoga postures, rejuvenating every system in the body, and promoting a unique perspective on the world. It is best learned initially with the guidance of a qualified yoga teacher.

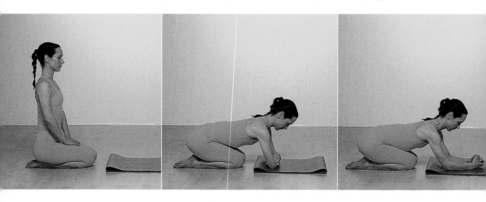

1 Kneel on the floor with your hands on your thighs. Place a folded nonslip mat in front of you. Inhale.

2 On an exhalation, bring your elbows to the mat, shoulder-distance apart. Push them into the mat.

3 Keeping your elbows still, interlock your fingers and rest your wrists on the mat. Roll your shoulders back and down.

TAKE CARE
Avoid if you have HBP, heart disease, glaucoma, a detached retina, other problems with your eyes or ears, congestion, or neck problems, if you are very overweight, or if you are menstruating.

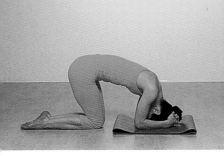

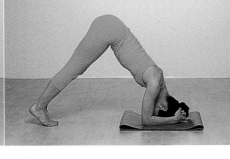

4 Bring the crown of your head to the floor and cradle the back of your head in the palms of your interlocked hands. Inhale.

5 On an exhalation, lift shoulders back and down away from your ears. Tuck toes under and straighten your legs, so you feel your weight resting now on your elbows and forearms. Lift your buttocks high.

6 Keeping the weight on your forearms and your shoulders away from your ears, begin to tiptoe your feet toward your head. Be aware of the shift in your center of balance as the feet come closer to your head. Sense that your spine is becoming vertical as the tailbone moves to align above the head. Breathe easily. ▶

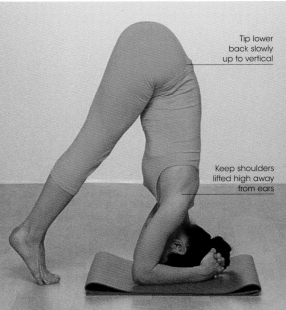

Tip lower back slowly up to vertical

Keep shoulders lifted high away from ears

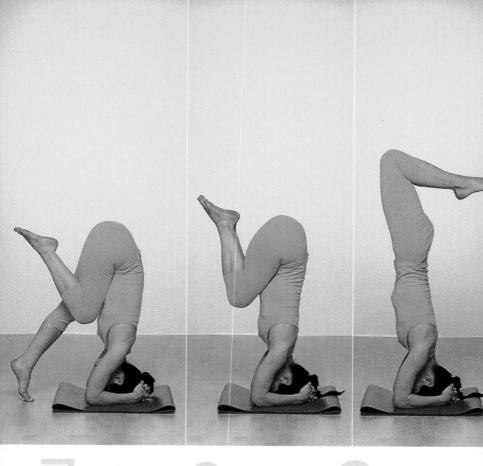

7 At the point when you feel the weight of your body shifting, pick one foot up from the floor, keeping the knee tucked in. Breathe freely like this.

8 Pick up the other foot. Stay in this position with the knees tucked in while you breathe easily and adjust yourself to the inversion.

9 When you feel confident and balanced, slowly lift the knees up, first to hip height, then above the hips. Allow the breath to flow easily.

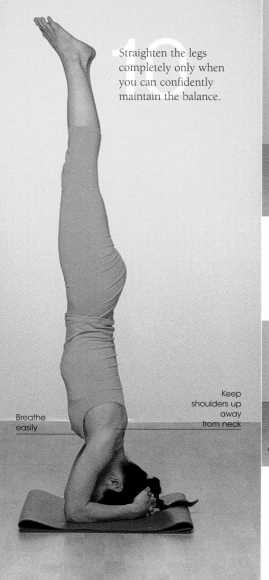

Straighten the legs completely only when you can confidently maintain the balance.

Breathe
easily

Keep
shoulders up
away
from neck

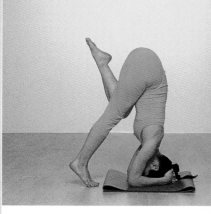

To come out of the posture, slowly tuck the knees down into the abdomen as in Step 8. Pause, then lower the feet, one at a time, to the floor.

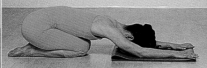

Bring the buttocks back on to the heels. Exhale completely and rest in Hare (see p.438) with the forehead on the mat.

spinal twist

Restful and refreshing, this simple twist stretches the abdominals and helps relieve stiffness caused by prolonged sitting. It also opens the chest and promotes flexibility in the hips.

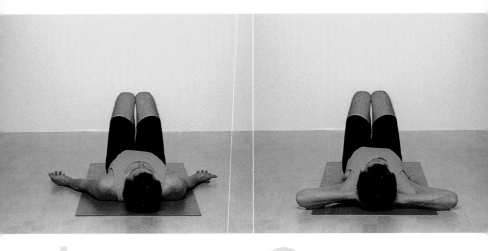

1 Lie on the floor with your knees bent and the soles of your feet flat. Keep the knees together and the back of your waist flat on the floor.

2 Clasp your hands behind the back of your head and let your elbows open out wide to the sides. Check that your chin is tucked in. Breathe into the abdomen.

On an exhalation, let your knees drop down toward the floor on the right-hand side, keeping them together as they are lowered down.

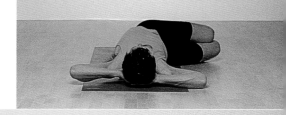

Once your knees reach the floor, turn your head to the left, breathing evenly. To come out of the pose, on an inhalation bring your head and knees back to the center. Repeat on the other side.

Let hips turn fully

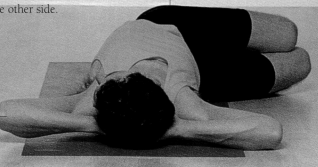

Keep elbows down

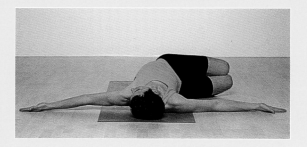

ALTERNATIVE

If your elbows do not reach the floor, take your arms out to the sides at shoulder level. Feel the contact between the shoulder blades and the floor. Keep chest open.

spinal twist 2

This pose has the same benefits as Spinal Twist (see p.454), stretching the abdominals and relieving stiffness caused by prolonged sitting. It also frees blocked energy in the shoulders and hips.

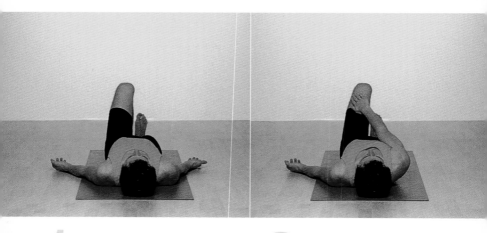

1 Lie on the floor with your legs stretched out, your knees and ankles together, and your arms stretched out to the sides, palms facing up. Bend your left knee and tuck the toes of your left foot under the back of your right knee.

2 Move your right arm across your body and place the palm of your right hand on your left thigh just above the knee. Breathe into the abdomen.

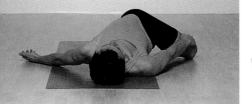

3 On an exhalation, allow your left knee to move across the body to drop down toward the floor. Once the knee reaches the floor, let it rest there, with your hand on top.

4 Turn your head to the left and breathe evenly in the pose for a few breaths. To come out of the pose, on an inhalation bring your head and left knee back to the center. Then repeat on the other side.

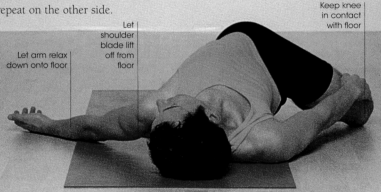

Keep knee in contact with floor

Let shoulder blade lift off from floor

Let arm relax down onto floor

ALTERNATIVE

To work the shoulder girdle more strongly, practice maintaining contact between the shoulder blades and the floor. This will probably mean that your knee will not reach the floor, so hold it in position with your hand.

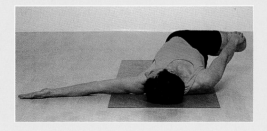

breathing
practices

The following breathing practices can be practiced on their own to improve your awareness of the breath, but they are particularly useful as preparatory practices before meditation (see p.470).

The breathing practices described here will help improve your breath awareness and encourage calmness and mental clarity. They are generally practiced after doing some yoga postures or simple stretching. Physical movement helps loosen up the body, so that it is easier to be relaxed during the breathing practices. Breath awareness is the crucial first step toward moving your attention within and learning to observe thoughts, feelings, and patterns of behavior.

Incorporating a mudra

You might like to use a mudra, or hand gesture, in conjuction with one of the breathing practices to improve its effectiveness. There are many mudras used in yoga practice. Two – the Gesture of Consciousness and the Gesture of Knowledge – are shown on pp.468–469. They also help to remind you of the link between the individual and universal consciousness – that we are all interconnected, never unsupported.

When you are familiar with Alternate Nostril Breathing (see opposite), try visualizing the movement of the breath without using the hands whenever you need to center yourself. Called Psychic Triangle Breathing, this can be useful when you need to re-establish confidence in a public place.

Stoking the Fire (see p.460) and Shining the Skull (see p.461) are best learned with a teacher. If you have any problems, be sure to seek help.

alternate nostril breathing

Breathing through alternate nostrils has a balancing effect on the mind, body, and emotions. Begin by observing the breath and then practicing the complete breath (see p.387). Do several rounds.

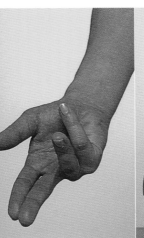 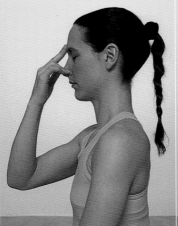 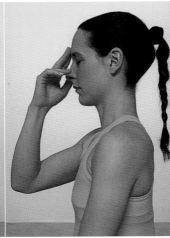

1 Sit comfortably. Lift the breastbone and relax the shoulders. Fold the little finger of the right hand into the palm. Keep the index and middle fingers straight and let the tip of the ring finger be opposite the thumb.

2 Raise your right hand to your face. Rest the index and middle fingers of the right hand between the eyebrows. Close the left nostril with your ring finger and breathe in through the right nostril.

3 Close the right nostril with the thumb and open the left. Breathe out through the left nostril, then breathe back in through it. Close the left nostril, open the right, and breathe out through that. This completes one round.

stoking the fire

This practice, which should be done on an empty stomach, develops great power in the abdominal muscles, promoting excellent digestion, increasing vitality, and helping to overcome depression and lethargy.

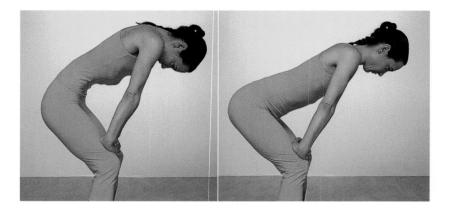

1 Stand with the feet hip-width apart. Bend the knees slightly and rest the heels of your hands on the thighs. Breathe evenly. Extend each inhalation and exhalation, so that you can feel the abdominal muscles "squeezing" the exhalation out. At the end of the next breath out, do not breathe in. Squeeze the muscles in a little tighter.

2 Release the muscles, letting the belly flop forward. Then pull the abdominal muscles sharply back in, and release them. Repeat, squeezing in and letting go of the muscles until you need to breathe in.

TAKE CARE
• If you experience dizziness or breathlessness, stop, take a break, then try more slowly and less forcefully. • Avoid if you have HBP or epilepsy, during menstruation, or if both nostrils are congested.

shining the skull

Like Stoking the Fire (see opposite), this practice should only be done on an empty stomach. It develops great power in the abdominal muscles, aids digestion, and increases vitality. Above all, it promotes clarity of mind.

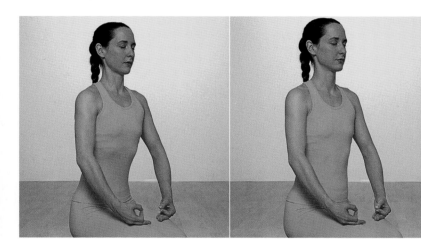

1 Kneel with the hands on the knees in the Gesture of Consciousness (see p.468). Feel the movement of the abdomen as you breathe in and out. At the end of an inhalation, draw the abdominal muscles in quickly and forcefully. This expels the air through the nose; the exhalation is felt and heard as the air leaves the nostrils.

2 Immediately allow the abdomen to release into softness, so that the inhalation happens all by itself. Repeat three to five times.

TAKE CARE
The same as for Stoking the Fire (see opposite).

humming breath

Humming breath is an antidote to stress, anger, and anxiety. It also induces a profound sense of calm, lowers blood pressure, and relieves insomnia. It strengthens the voice and promotes a relaxing inner peace.

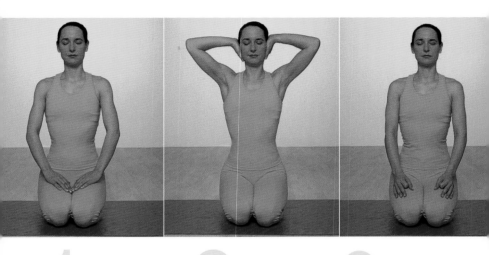

1 Sit comfortably with a straight spine in whichever of the sitting postures you prefer – Thunderbolt (see p.426) is a good basic position. Close your eyes and establish a complete breath (see p.387).

2 As you inhale, bend the elbows and draw them out wide at shoulder height. Block your ears with the heels of your hands. Keep the mouth closed, jaw relaxed, and teeth slightly apart as you breathe out, resonating a deep soft humming sound.

3 Allow the sound to fade at the end of the exhalation. Breathe normally. This is one round. Repeat five times. Keep your hands in position throughout. At the end of the last round, rest your hands in the Gesture of Knowledge (see p.469).

breath balancing

This practice promotes even breathing, aids digestion, and is a fast and effective way to center yourself.

Just a couple of minutes of breath balancing creates a calm and attentive frame of mind.

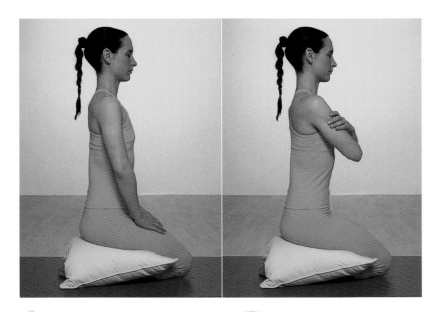

1 Sit on your heels with a straight spine. If this is uncomfortable, place a pillow between the buttocks and heels. Lower the shoulders away from the ears. With the hands resting on the thighs, watch the breath for seven rounds as you establish a complete breath (see p.387).

2 When the breath is rhythmic, tuck the right thumb high into the left armpit and the left thumb into the right armpit. Close the eyes. Be aware of a triangular pattern of breath, as the air flows into the nostrils and up the sides of the nose to the tip of the triangle between the eyebrows.

invocation of energy

Also known as "the peace gesture," this is an effective way of increasing vitality, trust, and confidence. The practice involves synchronizing the breath with arm movements. It is a symbolic giving and receiving of energy, which creates a powerful sense of tranquility and acceptance.

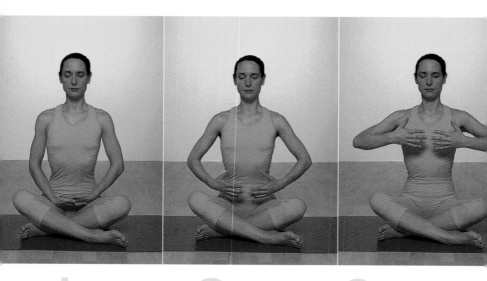

1 Sit comfortably with your legs crossed. Close your eyes. Cup your hands and rest them, palms facing upward, in your lap. Breathe evenly for three rounds.

2 As the abdomen begins to expand on the next inhalation, separate the hands and move them up to a little in front of the abdomen, tips of the fingers pointing toward each other.

3 As the ribcage begins to expand on the next inhalation, lift your hands up to just in front of your chest, until they are level with your nipples.

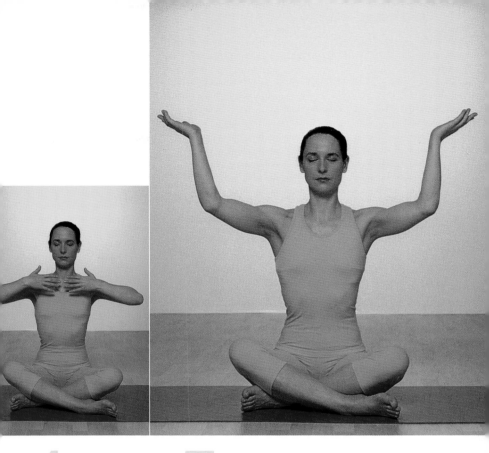

At the next inhalation, feel the top of your lungs expand as you raise your hands up to the level of the collarbones.

Hold your breath in your lungs as you open out your arms and turn your palms to face up. Remain in this position for as long as you can comfortably retain the breath. On the exhalation, gradually move the hands back down to the lap. Relax and breathe normally.

concentration
practices

Concentration practices develop mental focus, which is one of the key foundations of self-confidence. They also improve memory and can relieve anxiety, depression, and insomnia.

concentrated gazing

This practice begins by providing an external point of focus, and then shifts the attention to the after-image, which appears in the mind's eye. Withdrawing your attention to the internal world is a crucial step in acquiring the attentive self-awareness and quiet interior focus necessary to building self-esteem.

Use a comfortable seated position, such as Thunderbolt (see p.426), and place a candle at arm's length in front of you so that its flame will be precisely at eye level. With your head, neck, and spine aligned, place your hands in the Gesture of Knowledge (see p.469). Establish a rhythmic complete breath (see p.387) as you relax in your chosen seated posture.

Gradually increase the length of time you can gaze at the candle without blinking. Take it easy, and never strain the eyes. If you find that you become agitated by the rapidity or the nature of the thoughts and images passing through your mind, stop the practice and seek advice from a yoga teacher who has experience of its effects.

Developing mental focus and concentration takes time and patience, so, as you notice different thoughts or emotions, gently redirect your attention back to the object of your gaze.

PRACTICAL MATTERS
• Remove eyeglasses or contact lenses before starting the practice.
• Make sure the room is not drafty; otherwise, the flame of the candle will flicker and be distracting.

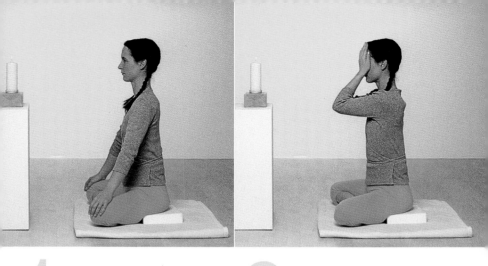

1 Let your gaze come to rest steadily on the flame at the tip of the candle wick. Allow your eyes to fix their gaze on this point without blinking or moving. Focus the awareness so completely on the flame that you are no longer consciously aware of your physical body.

Keep your gaze steady for as long as you can. When the eyes start to water or feel tired, gently close them. With the eyes closed, focus on the after-image of the candle flame that appears in the space in front of the closed eyes. Try to keep that image in place for as long as possible.

When the image begins to fade, open the eyes and look at the candle again. Keep the gaze focused for as long as you can, then close the eyes, focusing on the after-image of the candle. Repeat three or four times.

2 Rub your palms together vigorously until they feel warm, and cup the palms over your eyes. Feel the heat from the hands bathing the eyelids. Keeping the palms in place, open your eyes and look into the darkness within your cupped hands. When you are ready, lower your hands from your face.

TAKE CARE

• If you have epilepsy, do not focus on a candle flame, but instead use a fixed point, or an object or image of your choice.

• If you have severe eyestrain, myopia, astigmatism, or cataracts, use a black dot instead of a flame.

• If it is hard to focus on the flame at arm's length (because you are near- or far-sighted, for example), choose a distance at which you can focus easily, without straining the eyes.

using mudras

Mudras are traditional hand gestures that help you to center yourself. They help you quieten when you are feeling stressed, promoting a calm, meditative state of mind in which trust can be developed.

gesture of consciousness

Sitting cross-legged with your eyes closed, rest the backs of the hands on the knees or thighs, with the palms up. Bring the tip of each index finger to touch the tip of the thumb. Allow the rest of the fingers to be straight, but also relaxed and slightly apart from each other. Alternatively, tuck the tip of each index finger into the root of the thumb. You can also practice this mudra kneeling in Thunderbolt pose (see p.426).

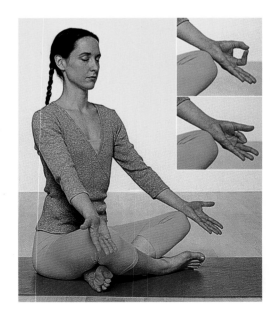

gesture of knowledge

Sitting with legs crossed (or in Thunderbolt – see p.426) and eyes closed, rest the palms of the hands on the knees or the thighs. Bring the tip of the index finger to touch the tip of the thumb. Alternatively, tuck the tip of each index finger into the root of the thumb. Let the rest of the fingers be straight but still relaxed and slightly apart from one another. This is a more inward-looking gesture than the Gesture of Consciousness, and is suitable for deeper exploration of your attitudes and beliefs.

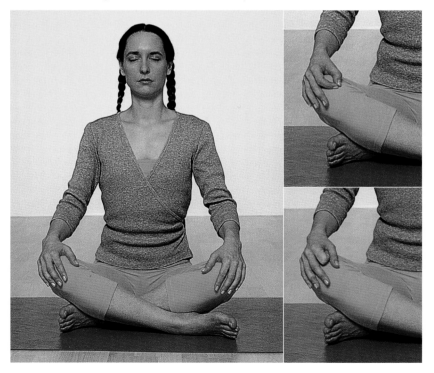

meditation

Meditation is a simple but profound practice that can bring about a state of focused attention and peace. Practiced often, it can teach you to observe and understand your thoughts and emotions.

inner silence meditation

This meditation practice takes about 15 minutes to complete. Sit in a comfortable position and close your eyes. Establish a Full Yogic Breath (see p.387). Rest your hands in the Gesture of Consciousness (see p.468).

PRACTICAL MATTERS
• Choose a time when you are certain that you will remain undisturbed for at least 15 minutes.
• Choose a room (or space outside) that is quiet, uncluttered, and not cold or drafty.
• Choose a posture – sitting in a chair, or sitting or kneeling on the floor – that you will be able to sustain easily for some time.

Let your awareness be with the sense of hearing. Listen to all the sounds. Start by bringing your attention to the loudest, then gradually draw the focus of your awareness in closer until you attend only to the quietest, closest sounds. Be aware of the sound of your own breath as it comes in and goes out.

Now shift the focus of your attention to the sense of touch. Become aware of the sensation of the breath passing into and out of the nostrils. Feel the cooler air coming in and the warmer air going out. Be aware of the different textures and temperatures that you can detect through the sense of touch. Sense if there is any difference between what you can feel on covered and uncovered skin. Then return to feeling the passage of air in the nose.

Now give your full attention to the sense of smell. Be aware of any odors and aromas around you. Then shift your attention to the sense of taste. Be aware of the tongue inside the mouth. Notice if there are sweet, salty, bitter, hot, or astringent tastes. Give the sense of taste full attention.

Now focus your attention on the sense of sight. Look into the closed eyelids and be aware of whatever you may see there. Are there any colors or shapes? Are there patterns, or movement? Just blackness?

Now spend a few moments simply watching the patterns of your own thoughts as they arise and pass away. Sit and wait for the first thought, watch it until it passes away, and then wait for the next thought to arrive. Do not get caught up with your thoughts or try to follow them.

After a little while, return your attention to the sense of hearing, and become aware of the intimate sound of your own breath. Allow that breath to get a little louder, and use the sound of that breath as a bridge back to becoming aware of other sounds in the room. Then widen your awareness until you are aware of sounds out in the wider world. When you are ready, open your eyes.

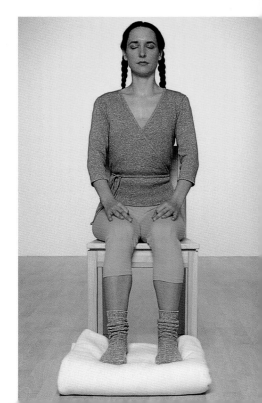

relaxation

Relaxing at the end of a yoga session gives the body and mind a chance to absorb the benefits of your practice. Set aside 20 minutes and follow the Deep Relaxation practice described below.

deep relaxation

This is a shortened version of one of the most powerful systematic approaches to profound relaxation. The Sanskrit for this practice is *yoga nidra* with *sankalpa*, which translates as "yogic sleep with affirmation." In fact, it is only the body that sleeps while the mind remains alert.

Lie on the floor in Corpse pose (see opposite). Close your eyes and establish 11 rounds of the complete breath (see p.387). Feel yourself settling the body into a state of stillness. Become aware of the points of contact between body and floor.

Make a resolve to let the body take deep rest, while the mind remains alert and attentive. Then prepare to carry the mental attention around the body, visiting each part of the body in turn, as if the light of the mind's attention were to come to shine briefly on each body part.

Keeping absolutely still, now bring the mental attention to touch each part of your body in turn. Choose a circuit that you can remember and that covers every part of the body. Try scanning down from top to bottom, or working clockwise around the body, or from the edges to the center.

When you have touched each part of the body in turn with your mental attention, bring the focus of your awareness back to the rhythm of the complete breath. Count 27 rounds of this, beginning at 27, and counting down to zero. If you lose count, start again.

When you get to the end of the last round of the complete breath, return to the resolve to let the body take deep rest, while the mind remains alert and attentive. Sense that the body is fully rested, and that the mind is alert and attentive. Then let your breath get a little noisier, until you can hear it clearly. Use the sound of the breath as the bridge back to a more everyday state of awareness. Stretch out through the fingers and toes, the hands and feet. Then stretch out through the whole body, roll over and sit up. When you feel ready, open your eyes.

Adding an affirmation

Once your are familiar with the sequence, you may want to make your own affirmation. Choose a simple, short, and positive statement about a direction you would like your life to take. Choose carefully, and make sure that you are happy with the affirmation before you work with it. When you feel you have the right affirmation, use it at the start and end of the relaxation practice.

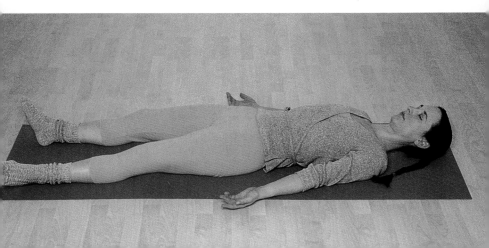

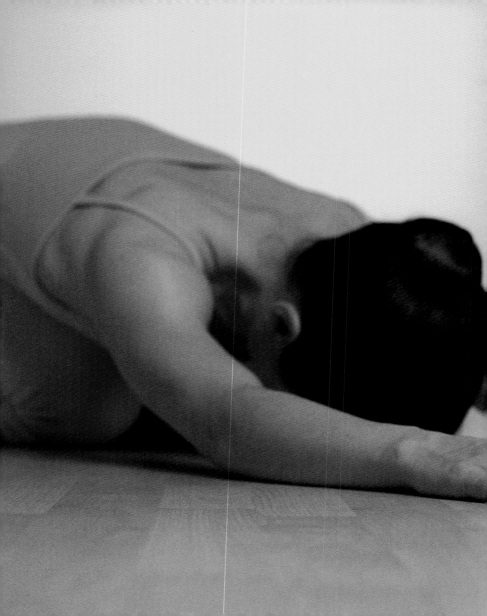

programs

The following seven programs will help boost your confidence in a variety of situations: before an exam or interview, during change and disruption, at times of self-doubt, when feeling panicky, when facing a challenge, and when you need to develop your self-worth.

1 pre-interview boost

Remaining confident and relaxed during an interview can be a challenge. This sequence, practiced before you set out for the interview, develops the energy and focus to approach your meeting positively. The final two practices can also be repeated on the way to the interview to maintain confidence and clarity of focus.

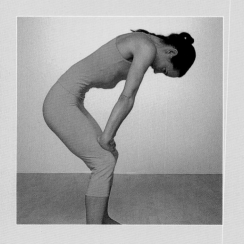

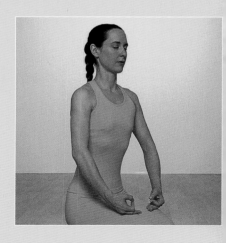

1 Stoking the Fire (see p.460)

2 Shining the Skull (see p.461)

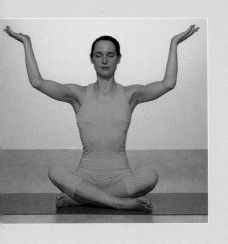

3 Invocation of Energy (see pp.464–465)

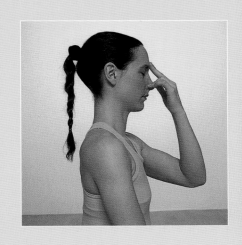

4 Alternate Nostril Breathing (see p.459)

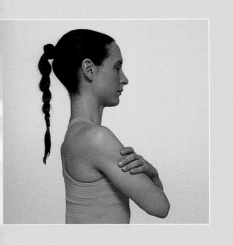

5 Breath Balancing (see p.463)

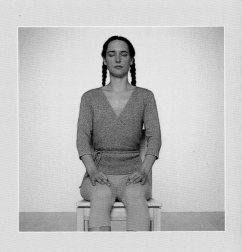

6 Inner Silence Meditation (see pp.470–471)

2 in times of
change

This sequence enhances your ability to adapt to changes in all aspects of life. To deepen the effect, practice the complete breath (see p.387) in Reverse Corpse and abdominal breathing (see p.387) in Hare. Use a focused gaze during Snake and Triangle. Complete the program with a period of Inner Silence Meditation (see p.470).

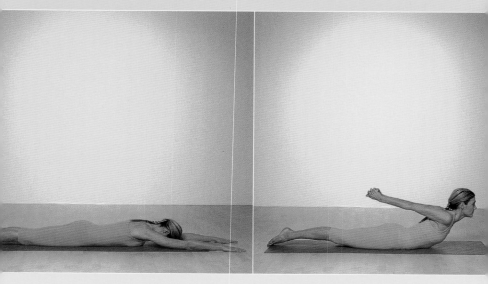

1 Reverse Corpse (see p.418)

2 Snake (see pp.416–417)

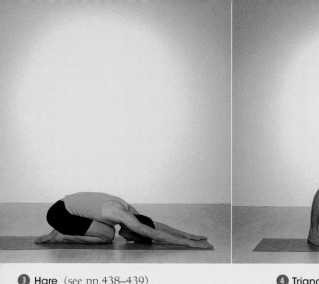

3 Hare (see pp.438–439)

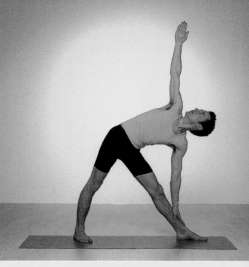

4 Triangle (see pp.402–403)

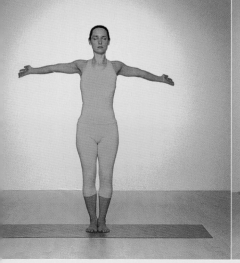

5 Arm Stretch 3 (see p.390)

6 Philosopher (see pp.428–429)

③ at low
moments

If you feel depressed, this program can help shift blocked energy, lift your spirits, and restore self-esteem. Begin with a few rounds of Stoking the Fire (see p.460). Allow the complete breath (see p.387) to flow through the Dancer, Tree, and Camel. Conclude with a stabilizing two minutes of Alternate Nostril Breathing (see p.459).

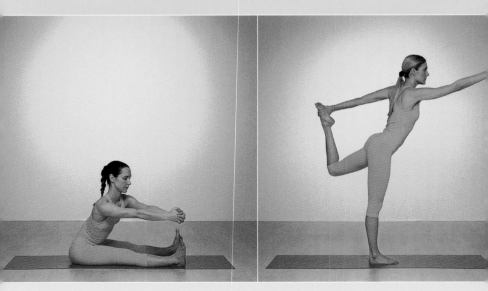

① **Stirring the Pot** (see pp.396–397)　　② **Dancer** (see pp.406–407)

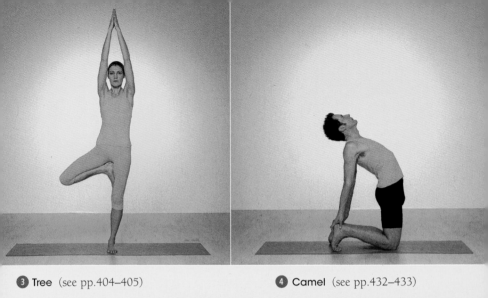

3 Tree (see pp.404–405)

4 Camel (see pp.432–433)

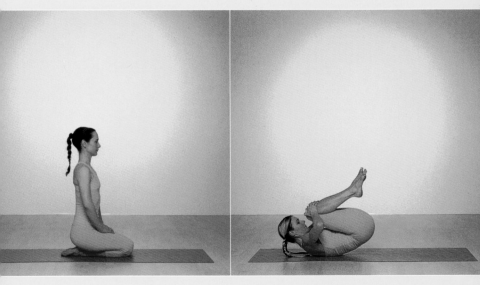

5 Thunderbolt (see pp.426–427)

6 Yogic Rock and Roll (see p.393)

4 for balance &
understanding

A balancing yoga program can help when your tolerance is challenged. Start with two minutes of the complete breath (see p.387). Then move through the postures, focusing on the breath. Complete the program with 27 rounds of Breath Balancing (see p.463) in Thunderbolt (see p.62), followed by Deep Relaxation (see p.472).

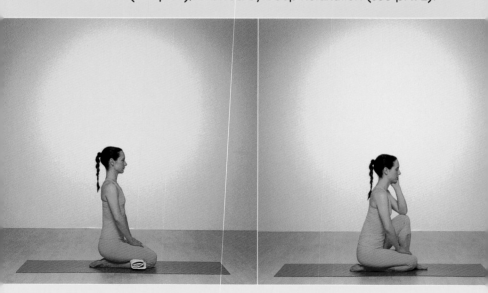

1 Thunderbolt (see pp.426–427)   **2** Philosopher (see pp.428–429)

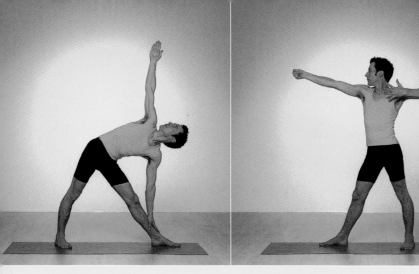

3 Triangle (see pp.402–403)

4 Bow and Arrow (see pp.400–401)

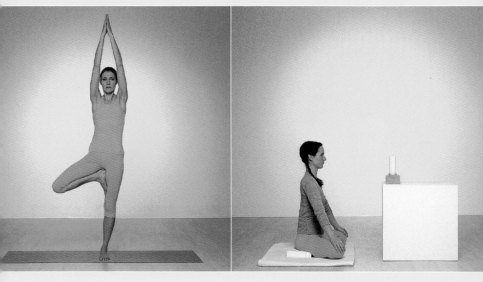

5 Tree (see pp.404–405)

6 Concentrated Gazing (see pp.466–467)

5 for stability & ease

This sequence brings the focus within, developing easeful self-acceptance. Begin with 11 rounds of the complete breath (see p.387) in Thunderbolt. Then hold each posture for at least seven abdominal breaths (see p.387). Complete the program with 11 rounds of Humming Breath (see p.462), followed by Deep Relaxation (see p.472).

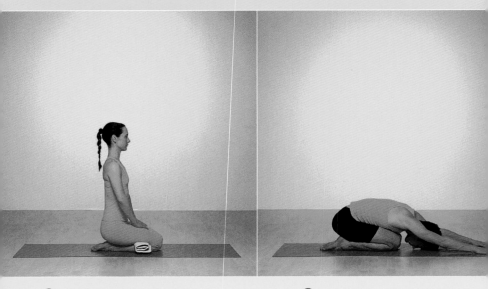

1 Thunderbolt (see pp.426–427)

2 Hare (see pp.438–439)

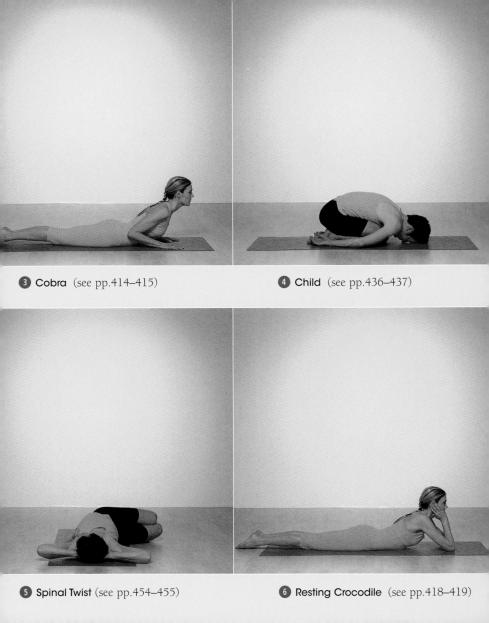

3 Cobra (see pp.414–415)

4 Child (see pp.436–437)

5 Spinal Twist (see pp.454–455)

6 Resting Crocodile (see pp.418–419)

6 for
courage

This program promotes strength and self-confidence to develop courage. Begin with seven rounds of the complete breath (see p.387). After Boat, do another 11 complete breaths before continuing with the postures. Conclude by quiet sitting in Thunderbolt (see p.426) and five rounds of Invocation of Energy (see p.464).

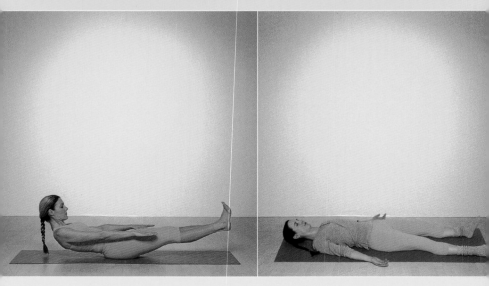

❶ **Boat** (see pp.408–409)　　　　❷ **Corpse** (see p.381)

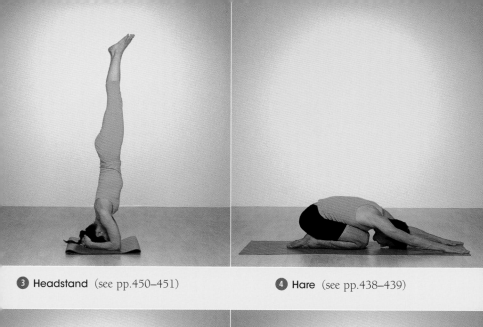

3 Headstand (see pp.450–451)

4 Hare (see pp.438–439)

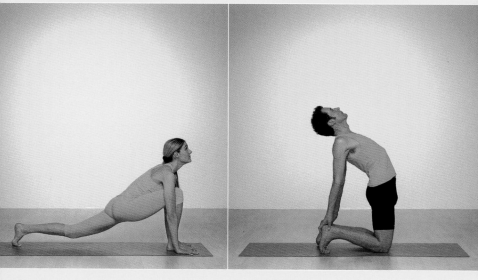

5 Lunge Warrior (see pp.412–413)

6 Camel (see pp.432–433)

7 to develop
self-worth

This program fosters compassionate self-acceptance and focused conviction. Take 11 rounds of the complete breath (see p.387) before you begin the postures, and another seven rounds after Boat. At the end of the program, do Inner Silence Meditation (see p.470), followed by Deep Relaxation (see p.472), using an affirmation.

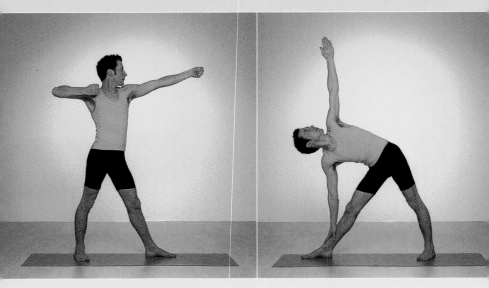

1 Bow and Arrow (see pp.400–401)　　　**2** Triangle (see pp.402–403)

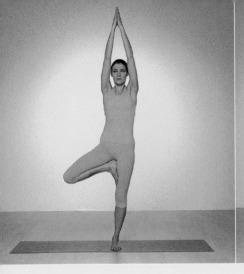

3 Tree (see pp.404–405)

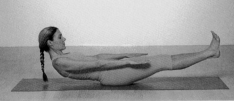
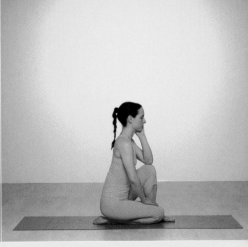

4 Boat (see pp.408–409)

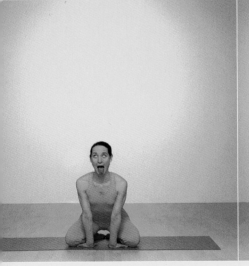

5 Roaring Lion (see pp.430–431)

6 Philosopher (see pp.428–429)

Index

Useful organizations

www.yogajournal.com
An interactive, in-depth yoga community website. Includes everything from postures to lifestyle advice, as well as a teachers' directory.

www.yogasite.com
A general source of information on yoga, with good links and a teachers' directory covering the United States, Canada, Australia, and other countries.

YOGA ALLIANCE
Tel: 888 921 9642;
Website: www.yogaalliance.org
Find an Yoga Alliance certified teacher or yoga center through this national Yoga Teacher's Registry

www.yogafinder.com
A directory listing yoga teachers, organizations, and events in the United States and other countries.

Acknowledgments

AUTHORS' ACKNOWLEDGMENTS
Peter Falloon-Goodhew:
Thanks to my teachers and students, especially Sheri Greenaway, Dr. Shrikrishna, and David Swenson; to Julie Bullock and Liz Taylor for help with the text; to Dr. Robin Monro for entrusting me with *Yoga for Living*; to Jane and Anne-Marie for their tireless editorial and design work and for being such fun to work with, and to Nicky and Schroeder for surviving the past year.

Ruth Gilmore:
I wish to thank Dr. Robin Monro of the Yoga Biomedical Trust for inviting me to write this book, Peter Falloon-Goodhew for coordinating the project, my family for their patience, and all who, wittingly and unwittingly, have shown me the yogic path.

Uma Dinsmore-Tuli:
Thanks to my mother, for teaching me confidence and showing me yoga at the age of four. Gratitude for the patience of my husband and sons. Dedicated to the living legacies of all Swami Sivananda's disciples, who shine the light of yoga throughout the world, especially Paramahamsa Satyananda Saraswati. Om Namaha Shivaya.

PUBLISHER'S ACKNOWLEDGMENTS
Thanks to Catherine MacKenzie for original design assistance; Helen Ridge, Jane Simmonds, and Angela Wilkes for editorial assistance; Dorothy Frame for the original indexing; and Anna Bedewell for additional picture research.

Models: Emma Cato, Jean Hall, Lee Hamblin, Jane Kemlo, Jade Littler, Kelly Smith-Beaney, and Cate Williams.
Photographer's Assistant: Nick Rayment
Hair and Make-up: Hitoko Honbu (represented by Hers)
Studio: Air Studios Ltd
Yoga mats: Hugger Mugger Yoga Products, 1190 S Pioneer Road
Salt Lake City, Utah 84104
Tel: 800 473 4888;
Fax: 801 268 2629;
Website: www.huggermugger.com;
email: comments@huggermugger.com
Yoga props: Yogamatters Ltd, 32 Clarendon Road, London N8 0DJ.
Tel: 08888 8588;
Website: www.yogamatters.com;
email: help@yogamatters.com

PICTURE CREDITS
The publisher would like to thank the following for their kind permission to reproduce their photographs:
8: Getty Images/Anthony Marsland; 14: Getty Images/Ian McKinnell; 18: Getty Images/Gary Buss;133: Getty Images/Pete Turner; 138: Getty Images/Jaques Copean; 253: Retna Pictures Ltd/Jenny Acheson; 256: Photonica/Hans Bjurling; 373: Photonica/Mats Widen; 378: Getty Images/Justin Pumfrey.
All other images © Dorling Kindersley.
For further information see:
www.dkimages.com